Peter Mansfield has spent his entire adult life learning through teaching. After 18 years of short sight he discovered the Bates method and learned to see. Peter lives in Sussex where he divides his time between teaching, writing and dinghy sailing.

THE
BATES
METHOD

A complete guide to
improving eyesight naturally

Peter Mansfield

Illustrated by
Shaun Williams

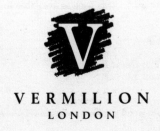

VERMILION
LONDON

First published by Macdonald Optima in 1992
Revised in 1995

1 3 5 7 9 10 8 6 4 2

Copyright © Peter Mansfield 1992, 1995

Peter Mansfield has asserted his moral right to be
identified as the author of this work in accordance with
the Copyright, Design and Patents Act 1988.

All rights reserved. No part of this publication may be
reproduced, stored in a retrieval system, or transmitted
in any form or by any means, electronic, mechanical,
photocopying, recording or otherwise, without the prior
permission of the copyright owner.

This edition published in the United Kingdom in 1996 by
Vermilion
an imprint of Ebury Press
Random House UK LTD
Random House
20 Vauxhall Bridge Road
London SW1V 2SA

Random House Australia (Pty) Ltd
20 Alfred Street, Milsons Point, Sydney,
New South Wales 2061, Australia

Random House New Zealand Limited
18 Poland Road, Glenfield,
Auckland 10, New Zealand

Random House, South Africa (Pty) Limited
PO Box 337, Bergvlei, South Africa

Random House UK Limited Reg. No. 954009

A CIP catalogue record for this book is available from the
British Library.

ISBN 0 09 181281 X

Printed and bound in Great Britain by
Mackays of Chatham, plc

Papers used by Vermilion are natural, recyclable
products made from wood grown in sustainable forests.

CONTENTS

PREFACE TO
THE SECOND EDITION

Since the appearance of the first edition I have been most
encouraged by the number of people who have written to
say how clear and helpful they have found the description
of the method after struggling unsuccessfully with some of
the older books. Apart from a few corrections, the main
changes here are revisions of the sections on eye diseases
and practising the method, and updates and corrections to
the information pages. I have also added some extra
appendices. Two of these relate to subjects about which I
am asked at least once a week, and the other covers the
implications of some recent research into vision development. Ideally I should have liked to incorporate this
information more fully into the text but it would have
involved rewriting half the book and since the conclusions
are still rather tentative, annexing it in this way seemed
the best solution.

PREFACE

This is a short book; nonetheless I have attempted to give a reasonably comprehensive and up-to-date account of the Bates method as practised in the UK.

Vision is a complex process. I hope I have managed, if not to simplify, at least not to over-complicate matters. Most writing on this subject has emphasised the use of exercises, and discussion has focused on the question of their effectiveness or otherwise. Over the years it has become clear that the methods proposed by Dr Bates work very well for some individuals, less well for others. In any discipline there is more to be learnt from 'failure' than from easy success, and it is from those who have persisted, despite finding the method less than easy, that teachers have learned where to go next. In this way our understanding of the meaning of the visual process continues to grow and the place of the Bates method in relation to other techniques of healing and re-education becomes clearer.

In one sense, the method is complete and self-contained and I regard it as essential that we maintain a tradition of teaching firmly based in the work of Dr Bates, and not arbitrarily revised to suit passing fashion or to 'buy off' criticism. However, it is also vital that the broad understanding of the visual process, as it involves mind, body and spirit, be not confined to the present handful of Bates teachers. As it touches on all areas of health and learning, so all health workers and educators need to take this understanding into account. Since Dr Bates wrote his book, billions of pounds/dollars and man-hours have been invested in optical and ophthalmic research, the main result of which seems to be more people than ever with faulty eyesight. Could it be, perhaps, time for a different approach?

ACKNOWLEDGMENTS

I am greatly indebted to all my teachers, colleagues and pupils for their patience and generosity. I must especially mention Anthony Attenborough and Miss E.B. Sage, together with the late Michael Ronan and Olive Scarlett, all of whom at various times helped my own vision and understanding. Also, everyone connected with the Bates College for keeping me on my toes, and, above all, Margaret Montgomery for her unflagging support and Clive Borst for putting me right about all the things I didn't know.

1
WHAT IS THE BATES METHOD?

The Bates method is an approach to the understanding and, where possible, the improvement of human vision. It originated with the work of the American ophthalmologist William H. Bates, and has been developed and refined by generations of his successors.

Dr Bates' book *Perfect Sight Without Glasses* describes how, through clinical observation, laboratory experiment and personal experience, he found that:

- Normal sight is inherently variable.
- Defective sight can get better as well as worse.
- Poor sight and eye disease are intimately related.
- Eyesight is an important indicator of mental, emotional and physical health.

From these discoveries he developed the practices and the underlying philosophy on which the present-day method is based.

Dr Bates' work can be thought of as comprising:

- A special theory of the operation of the eye.
- A general theory of seeing.
- A system of practical techniques for the improvement of vision.

The special theory is an attempt to describe the physical behaviour of the eye in forming the image of an object. The standard school-book explanation begs more questions than it answers, and Dr Bates felt justified in preferring a theory that explained more fully the facts he had observed.

The general theory of seeing, derived from Dr Bates' work, addresses human vision in a modern holistic context as an activity of mind, body and spirit, not of the eye alone. Seeing is considered as a skill that is learned and

1

practised from earliest childhood, while chronic disturbance of vision may be evidence of a lapse into bad habits and/or underlying disturbance of health. This framework for understanding visual problems makes it possible for many healing techniques not only to help improve vision but also to use vision as a guide to the improvement of health.

The practical technique evolved by Dr Bates approaches the problems of visual function through the experience of seeing. It gives a way of modelling the normal behaviour of the eyes and re-educating into normal habits of use. It is based on:

- Relaxation – awareness of the strain to see and acceptance of what is seen.
- Awareness and attention – developing conscious perception of what is seen.
- Memory and imagination.
- Integration of brain function.

This is not the only way to help poor sight, but it is often appropriate and highly effective, for the simple reason that a great deal of poor sight is due to bad habits of seeing, involving strain to see and lack of perception. In other cases it provides a practical way of thoroughly analysing the situation, identifying whatever help may be appropriate and monitoring progress.

WHO CAN BENEFIT?

The Bates method is valuable in every kind of visual disorder because it is based on restoring or ensuring the natural function of the eyes. Since it brings a unique insight to the relationship between eyes, brain and body, it also does good work in a range of conditions – physical, psychological and emotional – that might not normally be thought of as primarily visual in nature. Because it involves a particular understanding of learning processes, its principles make an important contribution to resolving all kinds of learning difficulty; for example my first experience in the method, beyond the improvement of my own sight, was to create a dramatically different and vastly more effective approach to music teaching.

Any limitation in the method stems not from the severity of the condition but from the personality involved. It is not a question of committing hours to the practice of exercises but of the willingness to change, to see differently.

I categorize potential pupils loosely into three groups. At one extreme are the desperate – those who have tried every avenue of medical science, have found them all wanting, and are facing blindness. Such challenging circumstances produce remarkable opportunities, to prove that nothing is impossible – Aldous Huxley in his time and Meir Schneider in ours are certainly good examples. However, not all the massively afflicted face their trials so heroically, and it needs to be remembered that lesser successes are valuable too.

At the opposite extreme, many people with perfectly good sight find themselves in glasses as a result of a temporary aberration, or even for no better reason than being told they need them by an authority. In such cases very little intervention is needed except to offer a different viewpoint – one that encourages people to trust their own perceptions more and to be more sceptical of the experts.

In between these two extremes are those who have perhaps worn glasses for some years, who have no special difficulty but who wish to take up the challenge of exploring sight as an opportunity for discovery and growth. For them the method is not just therapy; it is fun, fascination and, in every sense, *a way of seeing*.

Since the method emphasises conscious awareness and personal responsibility, it is sometimes asked 'How can very young children benefit?' The answer is, of course, that the child is in the care of its parents and it is their understanding, their decisions and their behaviour that will be the focus of attention until the child is able to take responsibility.

Difficult and spectacular cures of severe conditions are always newsworthy. Prevention, in contrast, is undramatic, un-newsworthy and may even be impossible to prove – one may only be able to infer that it has happened at all. Be that as it may, the Bates method sets out primarily to prevent the failure of sight, and to restore only as a last resort. Both activities, however, depend ultimately on our understanding of the process of seeing.

2
DR BATES AND
HIS WORK

William Horatio Bates was born in Newark, New Jersey, in 1860, and received his medical degree from the college of physicians and surgeons in 1885. He practised privately in New York City and attended at a variety of hospitals, including the Manhattan Eye and Ear Hospital and the New York Eye Infirmary. For five years he was an instructor in ophthalmology at the New York Postgraduate Medical School and Hospital, and at various times was medical adviser to school boards, including those of Rochester, NY, and New York City. From 1907 to 1922 he took outpatient clinics at the Harlem Hospital where he was assisted by Emily Liermann, who became his wife. Early in his career he contributed papers on his work to the major medical journals. After the publication of *Perfect Eyesight Without Glasses* in 1919, he continued to develop and promote his ideas through the journal *Better Eyesight*, and went on teaching and writing until his death in 1931.

RETINOSCOPY

The primary tool in much of Dr Bates' research was the retinoscope, an instrument of elegant simplicity, which allows direct assessment of the refraction of the eye. This had been established around the time of Dr Bates' birth, and the instrument was just coming into regular clinical use while he was a student.

He was evidently intrigued by the possibilities of this novel tool, and made it his speciality. Refining his technique through constant practice, he discovered that its scope was greater than had been realised – he became

5

The
Retinoscope   Subject

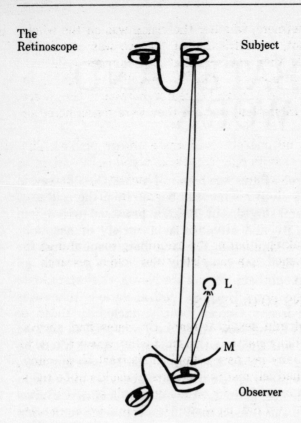

L

M

Observer

The retinoscope is a simple mirror with a small hole drilled through its centre. Light from the source L is reflected from the mirror M into the eye of the subject where it casts a shadow on the retina. The observer, viewing through the hole, rotates the mirror slightly from side to side and can tell from the movement of the shadow whether the eye is refracting accurately, or if it is long or short sighted.

particularly interested in observing animals and humans, children and adults, in normal activity in daylight, as opposed to the artificial surroundings of the consulting room. As his observations continued he began to suspect, then became certain, that the eyes of people seeing normally behaved differently from those who saw abnormally. Furthermore, whether the vision was on the whole normal or not, the refraction of the eye was constantly changing. He then realised that the changes reflected, among other things, the state of mind of the subjects, so that vision would always be nearer normal if they were relaxed and interested, worse if they were tense, bored or worried.

Why had no one observed these things before? The usual way of examining eyes was, as it still is, to work in a darkened room with the eyes dilated and partly paralysed with atropine drops. This is very convenient for clinical examination, but hardly the best way to get the eyes to act naturally. Dr Bates, by taking up retinoscopy almost as a hobby and taking it out of the examining room and on to the street, opened up a completely new field of research.

OBJECTIONS TO GLASSES

A thoughtful and sensitive man, Dr Bates had always found prescribing glasses an unsatisfactory answer to poor sight. Like many lay people (and in contrast to so many doctors), he had felt instinctively that it could not be right or natural in any sense for so many people apparently to have eyes that just did not work. Now he had evidence that this was not so.

Having observed that normal, as well as abnormal, sight was naturally variable, he noticed that in those who wore glasses the vision varied less and the eyes moved less freely. He reasoned that the movement and variation were important aspects of normal vision and were interfered with by glasses – evidence for his suspicion that glasses make vision worse. He realised, moreover, that in order to see through glasses it was necessary for the eyes to behave constantly in the same way as when they were fitted. 'Wrong' behaviour of the eyes was thus being rewarded and any attempt to act more normally was being punished. In order to escape from this topsy-turvy situation it would be necessary to stop wearing glasses and return the behaviour of the eye to normal. But how?

7

CENTRAL FIXATION

Dr Bates decided to regard the accuracy of the eye's focus (refraction) not as the starting point of the seeing process but as an end result. The key perhaps lay in the movements of the eyes: not the relatively large and slow 'pursuit' or tracking movements, but in the rapid vibrations that the normal eye makes continuously, even when ostensibly at rest. These *saccades*, as they are called, were the movements Dr Bates found most disturbed when the vision was poor, when glasses were worn or when there was evidence of any kind of strain. What did these movements have to do with clarity of vision? The answer lay in the structure of the retina.

The retina is the light-sensitive membrane within the

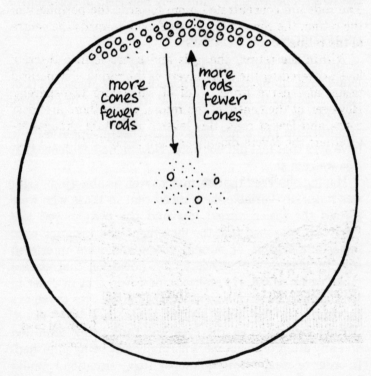

Distribution of rods o and cones · in the retina.

eye that collects visual images and transmits them to the brain. Whereas photographic film is equally sensitive over all its surface, the retina is constructed so that its sensitivity varies. There are two kinds of light receptor cells, known as *rods* and *cones* because of their approximate shapes.

- The *rods* are more sensitive to light, but give lower image resolution. They are most used in low-light vision and for general orientation. In photographic terms they are fast, monochrome (are sensitive only to black and white) and coarse grained.
- The *cones* are the opposite – fine grained, colour sensitive, but rather slow. They specialize in sharp resolution and colour definition, but require more light to operate.

The rods are concentrated more towards the periphery of the retina, the cones concentrated more towards the centre of the retina.

Within the retina, the rods and cones form a discrete layer, covered by the other layers of the retina – structural tissue and nerve fibres – all of which are transparent. However, at the centre of the retina, where there are most cones and fewest rods, this layered structure changes altogether; the layers disappear completely so that a small

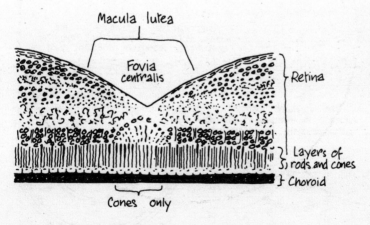

Section through the centre of the retina.

depression is formed, consisting solely of cone cells and their associated nerve structures. This, from its appearance, is known as the *macula lutea* (yellow spot). Even blood vessels do not appear in this area – tiny capillaries terminate in a wreath around the macula, but none cross it. At the centre of the macula itself is a tiny indentation, the *fovea centralis*, which contains nothing but closely packed cone cells.

The effect of this is to enable the fovea, under suitable conditions, to form a far more intense image than any other part of the retina, so that the precise centre of the field of vision is unmistakably defined. This minute area (less than a pinpoint) is so important that it has its own dedicated bundle of fibres within the optic nerve so that its signals can travel separately from those of the rest of the retina.

The macula lutea is thus one of the most extraordinarily interesting features of the human eye, yet, although it is described in every ophthalmic textbook, most are vague about its purpose and take little interest in it unless it happens to become diseased. Dr Bates, however, took a great deal of interest in it and discovered that the function of the fovea in relation to the rest of the retina was crucial to all the operations of vision.

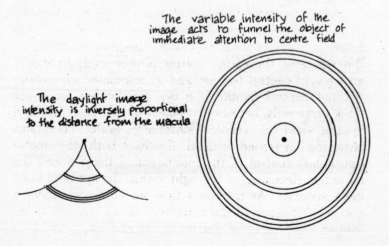

The variable intensity of the image acts to funnel the object of immediate attention to centre field

The daylight image intensity is inversely proportional to the distance from the macula

The point of fixation is the point to which attention is directed at any given moment. Central fixation, then, means that the point of immediate attention is always regarded directly by the fovea centralis. This does not imply that the eye should be fixed in the ordinary sense: on the contrary, in order for central fixation to be maintained, the eye must be constantly moving. Dr Bates found that the tiny eye movements he had observed in normal vision were essential to stimulate the fovea properly – according to his reasoning, if the eye stares fixedly, the fovea becomes no more sensitive than the surrounding retina. If this happens all kinds of aberrations of vision follow, simply because the eye literally loses its sense of direction.

The problem, therefore, is circular. Lack of central fixation obviously leads to poor vision, but poor vision also leads to loss of central fixation because those who do not see well either strain to see or stare blankly, not expecting to see, both habits tending to fix the eye rigidly. Wearing glasses confuses the situation as the glasses are adapted to the staring condition and provide clear vision, of a sort, without the benefit of central fixation. This encourages the unconscious belief that it is possible to see all parts of the field of vision equally clearly at once, re-inforcing the staring habit.

Staring, the attempt to see all parts of the field equally, could, so Dr Bates hypothesised, arise equally well from anxiety and greed to see, or from apathetic indifference. But whatever the cause, staring always leads to strain, with loss of central fixation and its associated movement. Without central fixation the eye can neither focus nor track accurately, because the object cannot be centralised in the field of vision. Conversely, under conditions favouring increased central fixation, both the motor (muscular) control of the movement of the eye and the refraction (focusing) of the light within the eye tend to be more accurate. At the same time an observer notices a marked difference in the movement of the eye, while the subject – the viewer – is able to discern that a small area

11

at the centre of the field of vision appears brighter and clearer than its immediate surroundings.

THE MECHANISM OF FOCUS

Having discovered vision to be variable, and having identified an important element of that variability, Dr Bates began to question the anatomical theories on which optical practice was based.

The traditional view

The mechanism by which the eye accommodates (changes focus) for different distances, together with many other visual topics, had been for centuries subject to much debate between competing theories. When Hermann von Helmholtz compiled his *Treatise on Physiological Optics*, his declared intention was to achieve a synthesis, to 'chart a path through the labyrinth'. Revealingly, in his preface we read

> Finally however, an effort had to be made to introduce law and order in this region and to rid it of the curious contradictions which have heretofore impeded progress. I have proceeded on the conviction that law and order, even if they are not fundamentally sound, are better than contradictions and lawlessness.

This may sound more like a Wild West sheriff than a scientist, but one can appreciate his intentions. However, impatience with contradictions can all too easily lead us conveniently to overlook facts that would otherwise disturb an established theoretical structure. Helmholtz meant his work to be the starting point for further research and new discoveries, instead of which it is today often used as a shield of dogma to hide a lack of curiosity and original thought. (It is a curious coincidence that the second volume of Helmholtz' work appeared in the year of Dr Bates' birth, while the second complete edition appeared in the year of his graduation.)

On the questions of refraction and accommodation,

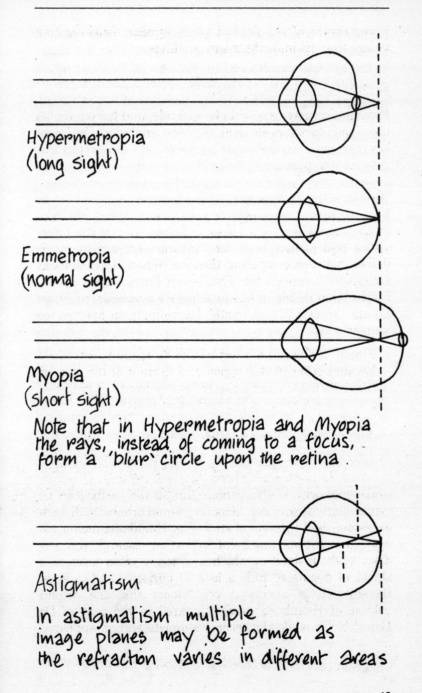

Hypermetropia
(long sight)

Emmetropia
(normal sight)

Myopia
(short sight)

Note that in Hypermetropia and Myopia
the rays, instead of coming to a focus,
form a 'blur' circle upon the retina.

Astigmatism

In astigmatism multiple
image planes may be formed as
the refraction varies in different areas

Helmholtz wholeheartedly adopted the views of the Dutchman Donders. Donders maintained that the shape of the eye was determined by accident of birth. It would grow, like every part of the body, according to the genetic programming, but otherwise its shape could not be varied. The shape and size of the eye alone determined its accuracy for distant vision. If the eye was just right (emmetropic), vision would be perfect. If it was too long (myopic), images would focus in front of the retina and one would be short-sighted. If it was too short (hypermetropic), the image would form behind the retina and one would be long-sighted. Astigmatism (confusion of focus) he considered to be due to a congenital deformity of the entire sclera (the outer layer of the eye) or of the cornea (the transparent part of the sclera, which forms the eye's 'window').

The adjustment of focus for near vision was attributed to the crystalline lens, which could be deformed by the action of the ciliary muscle that lies behind the iris (the coloured ring round the black pupil of the eye). Presbyopia – the failing of vision in old age – was explained as the lens hardening and refusing to change shape, as weakness of the ciliary muscle, or a combination of the two. This theory is extremely convenient for prescribing glasses, since it supposes that there is a 'true' refractive state of the eye,

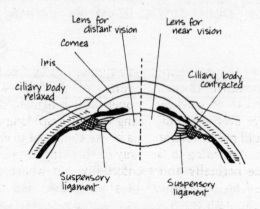

Accommodation according to Donders

which can be uncovered and accurately measured. It also sounds, on the face of it, neat and plausible, although the calculations involved are extremely complex and not neat at all.

Mathematics apart, Donders' theory has some interesting ramifications. It implies that vision can only be expected to be normal at one stage of growth. It is held to be normal and necessary for an infant to be long-sighted in order to grow into normality later; too little growth and one remains long-sighted, too much and the eye will elongate into incurable myopia. Bearing this in mind I have often wondered, since presumably the eyes grow at the same rate as the rest of the body, how the overgrown prodigies of American football and basketball can see anything at all.

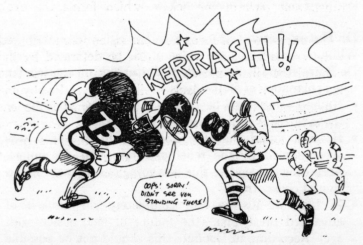

Just as the eye shape was supposed to be fixed, so the accommodative (focusing) range of the lens was only supposed to be used for 'proper' adjustment to distance. Under- or over-accommodating to 'cover up' long or short sight could not be tolerated as it was supposed to endanger the eyes. According to this way of thinking, a person who could see normally and comfortably, but whose optician diagnosed an error, would be given glasses and made to wear them, with threats of awesome consequences should he refuse.

Whether one inclines to believe in a creator or in the guiding hand of evolution, it seems extraordinarily slipshod to design a visual system that will not work in most cases; most second year engineering students could do a better design job. It has been blandly asserted nonetheless that the human eye was never intended for prolonged close-up use, and that the demands of civilisation have created a problem that civilisation and science must solve with optical glassware. In the interests of 'law and order', any facts that appeared to subvert this theory have been referred to as anomalies – curious, even amusing, but not significant – or, failing that, they would be ignored or denied – outlawed in fact. For their refusal to fit the all embracing theory they have, in the view of the authorities, lost their right to be considered facts.

Dr Bates' view

While never denying the value of his predecessors' work, Dr Bates found it necessary to go further in seeking the true explanation of all the facts.

- He had established beyond doubt that the accuracy of the eyes' focus could vary very considerably.
- He had found that the improvement of vision was accompanied by the relief of strain and discomfort. According to Donders this was going against nature and should *cause* strain.
- In his mid-40s he had completely rid himself of advanced presbyopia (the failure of near vision with age). According to Donders this should not be possible since presbyopia was supposed to involve irreversible physiological change.
- In laboratory work he used the retinoscope to demonstrate that accommodation (the change of focus from far to near) was induced by stimulus, not of the ciliary muscle, but of two of the external muscles of the eye – the inferior and superior obliques.

He expressed himself forthrightly:

A truth is strengthened by an accumulation of facts. A

working hypothesis is proved not to be a truth if a single fact is not in harmony with it. The accepted theories of accommodation require that a multitude of facts should be explained away. During more than thirty years of clinical experience, I have not observed a single fact that was not in harmony with the belief that the lens and the ciliary muscle have nothing to do with accommodation and that the change in the shape of the eyeball responsible for errors of refraction are not permanent.

Accommodation according to Dr. Bates

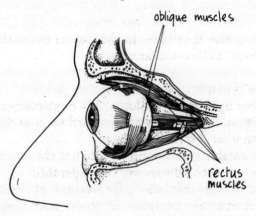

oblique muscles

rectus muscles

The rectus muscles act in concert to flatten the eyeball (for distant vision). The obliques lengthen it (for close vision).

His account of the facts as he saw them included the following:
- The eyeball is not fixed in shape, but flexible.
- The external muscles, which control the movements of the eye, also act in coordination to *control its shape*, and hence the focus both for distant vision and in accommodation. The action of the ciliary muscle in shaping the lens is of secondary importance.
- The primary function, determining accuracy both of movement and focus, is central fixation.
- Loss of central fixation is always due to strain. Poor

17

vision will be improved by encouraging central fixation, which will permit normal coordination of the muscles.
- Any direct attempt to see will intensify the strain and make the vision worse.
- Strain is not caused by poor sight: poor sight is caused by strain.

THE ROLE OF THE MIND

'We see very largely with the mind and only partly with the eyes.' (W.H. Bates, *Perfect Eyesight*)

The mechanics of vision – which muscles do what – although vital, are much less interesting than the electronics, the way in which the eyes receive direction from the mind.

In the ordinary way, the study of perception is treated as a branch of psychology and largely divorced from the physical study of the eyes. It has been commonly assumed that the eyes function automatically, and that the mind simply does its best with what it is offered. Dr Bates realised that this could not be so: perception must be *fed back* to direct the behaviour of the eyes. If an eye squints or wanders it is no use looking for the fault in the muscles. Likewise it is no use complaining that a short-sighted eye makes it difficult to perceive if lack of perception has created and maintains the short sight.

Very early in his work Dr Bates had observed that states of mind, emotions, preoccupations made a marked difference to vision. He also discovered clear links between vision, memory and imagination – not surprisingly, since memory, immediate perception and imagination are, so to speak, past, present and future aspects of the same process. Every perception is compared with memory (what went before?) and transformed in imagination (what/where next?) in order to translate into action – a movement or a focal adjustment of the eye.

The (MK. 1) Bates method

Based on these discoveries, Dr Bates began to develop a practical system of eyesight improvement. To the surprise of his patients, instead of prescribing glasses he began to set about teaching them to see by:

- Discarding glasses.
- Resting the eyes.
- Learning to focus the attention, while at the same time ...
- Avoiding efforts to see.
- Developing central fixation, directly through visual discrimination and indirectly through the experience of movement.

All this with extraordinary success in many cases.

PREVENTION VERSUS CURE

If poor eyesight could be cured it should be easier, not to say more satisfactory, to prevent it. Dr Bates spent a part of his working life visiting schools to test children's eyesight. Noticing variations in the results, he realised that practice in reading a test card could actually improve the vision.

Then, as now, a proportion of children could be relied on to develop abnormalities of vision in every school year. In Grand Forks, Dakota, with a school population of several hundred, Dr Bates found 6 per cent of the children myopic. Regular use of a daily drill with a test card reduced this to less than 1 per cent consistently over a six-year period. Similar programmes in other areas produced similarly good results. The drill that he devised was carried out in the classroom, the children sitting in their normal places, and took less than two minutes each day. 'Sometimes the results of the system were nothing less than astonishing – but in the end the board of education and the eyeglass specialists couldn't agree, and gradually the use of test cards for this purpose was dropped.' (Dr W.H. Bates *Perfect Eyesight Without Glasses*)

DR BATES AND HIS FOLLOWERS

Dr Bates' work naturally attracted a good deal of attention, not to say controversy. His opponents were and are those who will trust well-established theory rather than actual experience, or who would subject the method to a 'trial' in which it must work as instantly and invariably as glasses (which of course it doesn't) or be damned. Even those who supported Dr Bates, and who were on the whole enthusiastic about 'natural vision improvement', often seem to have had difficulty in understanding what he had in mind. His book is certainly difficult to read, not because of obscure or difficult language – he writes very plainly – but because of the challenge his ideas present to established patterns of thought.

His intention and hope was always that his discoveries would be accepted by his medical colleagues and be absorbed into standard practice. That is probably why he was rather casual about the training of other teachers – only a few learnt from him, and then in a rather *ad hoc* fashion by assisting in his clinic. Dr Bates seems hardly to have realised that he was creating a completely new discipline, trading an old branch of medicine for a novel departure in education. Had he invented new techniques in surgery or refraction, his colleagues would certainly have taken them up, but, whereas he was willing and able to give up those tools to become a teacher, the others were not; in fact they almost certainly could not understand what he was trying to do.

Ironically, although the name W.H. Bates is not popular in optomedical circles, a number of practices in modern optometrics and orthoptics have been assimilated from the more mechanical aspects of Dr Bates' work. As yet, however, medicine has failed to appreciate the subtlety of his understanding of the psychological aspects.

The realisation of what Dr Bates taught and practised is work, not for a medical technician, but for an educator, and so the work has passed out of medical hands. Very few teachers of the Bates method now have medical or optical training and the method is none the worse for that. The method is at present best established in India, the USA and the UK. In the Indian schools, under Dr Agarwal, Dr Bates' understanding of vision has been absorbed into a tradition embracing yoga meditation, homoeopathy and ayurvedic medicine. In the USA, most Bates activity derives directly or indirectly from the work of Aldous Huxley's teacher, Margaret Darst Corbett, who trained many teachers. The Corbett group developed many refinements and innovations, particularly in the area of binocular vision. Some US teachers have made a link between eyesight work and Reichian psychotherapy, leading to offshoots such as Radix and Visionetics. In 1954 the 'Bates-Corbett' school was badly disrupted by the prosecution of Clara Hackett for allegedly practising medicine without a license. (Reich also suffered very badly in the general climate of intolerance of unorthodoxy.) This was clearly misguided since the Bates teacher, in teaching people to use their eyes, is no more pretending to medicine than the piano teacher who teaches people to use their ears and hands, but it did restrict the growth of the work for a time. Currently the educational basis of the work is accepted in most states and vision education, in various forms, is quite widely available. In England there have always been a small number of teachers. The first were Kate and Ethel Beswick, and Captain C.S. Price. Price and Ethel Beswick had both visited Dr Bates at the Harlem clinic in the early 1920s and practised in London from about 1926. The Beswicks trained other teachers, including Olive and Marie Scarlett, who in turn set up a clinic and training school together with Madeleine Fousset, who had also been taught by Dr Bates. Survivors and descendants of that school have formed the main body of vision educators in the UK since that time, although the number of active teachers has rarely reached double figures. There is currently a real growth of interest which is materialising as a rapid rise in the number of teachers, as well as those making use of the method for themselves. Teachers in other countries are mostly either US or UK trained.

3
SEEING IN CONTEXT

We all understand new ideas according to our previous experience. The Bates method has been taken up by many people of different backgrounds, who have understood it in their own ways, with the result that Dr Bates and his ideas have been re-interpreted according to taste in terms of diet and physical exercise, yoga, psychotherapy (Freudian, Adlerian, Jungian and, especially, Reichian), mechanical engineering and even army drill. I do not claim to be an exception, and naturally my own account of 'the truth' of what Dr Bates had to say reflects my own background and interests. The most I can urge as to its objective correctness is that it is broadly supported by most of the people whose opinions I respect.

As I understand it, Dr Bates' approach to seeing is broadly of a piece with the tradition of thought expressed in the *Tao de Ching* and developed through centuries of Buddhism – that of doing through non-doing. This way of thinking has informed not only spiritual teaching but also many successful approaches to thoroughly practical problems over the last century or two. The best known exponent of recent years has been Timothy J. Gallwey, whose Inner Game series has turned a philosophical principle into a marketing triumph. Earlier, less well-known individuals such as the Swiss psychologist Roger Vittoz and the American pianist Luigi Bonpensière had applied the non-doing principle, expressed in very similar terms, to the treatment of neurosis and neurasthenia, and to the problems of virtuoso performance, respectively. The philosopher and novelist, Aldous Huxley, who learned the

Bates method from Margaret Corbett, explored the whole field in his book *The Perennial Philosophy*, and drew out the broad implications of Dr Bates' work, together with a useful practical account, in *The Art of Seeing*. Huxley's friend Olive Brown developed a practice, described in her book *Your Innate Power*, which draws out very distinctive insights from the work of Dr Bates, of Dr Vittoz and of F.M. Alexander.

In Britain, at least, Alexander's work has always been an important external reference point for Bates teachers, most of whom have considerable practical experience of the Alexander Technique. In particular, the language Alexander evolved to describe the learning process is as useful to describe Dr Bates' concept as his own.

F.M. ALEXANDER AND HIS TECHNIQUE

F.M. Alexander (1869–1955) probably contributed more than anyone else this century to our understanding of the relationship between mind and body. The Alexander Technique, as it is usually taught, concentrates on modifying the behaviour of the body in activity, to avoid self-inflicted damage and/or to enhance performance. Underlying the technique is a principle of great insight and subtlety which has much wider applications.

Alexander taught that:

- Mind and body are one. The division of activity into physical and psychological components is arbitrary and meaningless – one must address the human organism as a *psychophysical whole*.
- The *use* of the psychophysical unit will determine its level of function in the short term and hence its condition in the long term, i.e. prolonged *misuse* will cause chronic malfunction and hence physical deterioration in the long run.
- The treatment or exercise of any specific part is likely to be helpful only in so far as there is proper use of the organism as a whole. Specific work that adversely affects the *overall* use is invariably harmful.

- Use is largely determined by *habit* and by one's perception of what is happening, both of which may be faulty.

This last point needs amplification. Habit and perception shape each other in such a way that an act that is familiar, no matter how great the misuse involved, is likely to feel *right*, whereas an unfamiliar act is likely to feel *wrong*, even if the use is good. When misuse is present, therefore, attempts to learn or change will always be subverted because, in attempting either to imitate a model or to carry out instructions, one is always likely to base the critical judgment as to whether one is 'doing it right' on the habitual feeling, which will always prefer the familiar, i.e. the very thing one is trying to change. In short we are all in the same predicament as Lewis Carroll's Alice: 'wandering up and down and trying turn after turn, but always coming back to the house, do what she would. Indeed once, when she turned a corner rather more quickly than usual, she ran against it before she could stop herself.' (*Through the Looking Glass and What Alice Found There.*)

The problem is aggravated by a tendency to try to do things 'on the cheap', to go for an immediate result without considering the overall use or the long term-cost. Alexander called this '*end-gaining*'. The only solution was to reason out the '*means whereby*' a thing can be done with the most satisfactory use and to stick to it, regarding the feeling as to right and wrong with the greatest scepticism and judging strictly by results.

Since the habits of doing and their associated feelings are unreliable, any attempt to gain a given end directly will lead to misuse. One therefore has to act indirectly – to bring about the result through non-doing. To bring this about one must learn inhibition, i.e. to recognise the habitual response to a given stimulus and to prevent it, as a first step towards allowing the body to work differently. 'A little provoked, she drew back, and after looking everywhere for the Queen (whom she spied out at last, a long way off), she thought she would try the plan, this time, of walking in the opposite direction. It succeeded beautifully' (*Through the Looking Glass and What Alice Found There.*)

This all aligns precisely with Dr Bates' way of thinking and working. Strain, in Dr Bates' parlance, equates to misuse and end-gaining in Alexander's. Since relaxation is always discussed in relation to strain, it is clear that Dr Bates' conception of relaxation was not a state of inert collapse, of which Alexander was rightly critical, but an equivalent to Alexander's idea of balanced use achieved through inhibition and the means whereby principle. Aldous Huxley understood and expressed this very clearly, but others, unfortunately including Alexander himself, seem to have missed the point.

'Recognising and inhibiting an habitual end-gaining response to a familiar stimulus, substituting a reasoned means-whereby the end may be achieved' is an awful mouthful, but it is a good description of how to behave when confronted with a test card (see pages 150–53). At any rate, thinking about it in these terms puts the whole matter in a rather different light from the usual idea of 'doing eye exercises', and the further from that idea one can get, the better.

HOMOEOPATHY

Another reference point that has been invaluable to myself and others in understanding and applying Dr Bates' teaching is homoeopathy. Since its initial development by the German doctor Samuel Hahnemann (1755–1847), and despite its detractors, homoeopathy has grown to a pre-eminent place in world medicine. Ironically, during Dr Bates' lifetime, the USA boasted some of the world's leading homoeopathic schools and hospitals, but since he trained and practised in the allopathic institutions he probably had no contact with homoeopathic thought or practice. Had he done so, history could have been different in respect of the development of his ideas and of their reception.

As in the case of the Alexander Technique (or, indeed, the Bates method) there is a useful provisional distinction to be made between philosophy and practice. Homoeopathy does not consist in giving potentised medicines any more than the Bates method consists in doing eye exercises. In both cases the practice is underpinned by an attitude towards health and sickness that informs and sustains it. In the long and distinguished history of homoeopathy, many brilliant minds have applied themselves to expressing this attitude in clearly formulated statements of principle, many of which are directly helpful when thinking about the visual process, the meaning of poor sight and the way to go about improving it.

Some homoeopathic principles are as follows:
- Disease is a disturbance of the 'vital force'.
- Symptoms are the outward signs of the body's attempt to free itself from disease.
- The nature and order of appearance of symptoms is the best guide to cure.
- Suppressing symptoms will not cure disease but will drive it inward and make it worse.
- A symptom may affect a particular organ, but disease is of the whole.
- To achieve cure one must always work with the totality of symptoms – physical, emotional and mental. Treating an isolated symptom is likely to be suppressive.
- In a true cure, symptoms will disappear in the reverse order of their appearance.
- The body is self-healing. The aim of any treatment is to remove obstacles and stimulate the body's own healing power (vital force), using the minimum intervention.

Homoeopathic philosophy also makes useful distinctions between predisposition (constitutional and hereditary) and causation in disease; and between *exciting* causes (those that 'trigger' a disease process) and *maintaining* causes (that prevent cure, although they would be insufficient to excite disease).

Homoeopathy was the first modern discipline to insist on the unity of mind and body and on the importance of treating any conditions on the totality of symptoms. The parallels with both Dr Bates' and Alexander's thinking are striking, and the homoeopathic language, like Alexander's, can be applied to bring a certain precision to the discussion of visual problems.

If poor sight is symptomatic of emotional or mental disturbance, correcting vision with glasses clearly amounts to suppressing a symptom while disregarding the cause. Many people assume that poor sight is hereditary; we might cautiously speak of an hereditary predisposition, which will involve mental and emotional, as well as physical, characteristics. For poor sight actually to develop, though, we require an exciting cause, perhaps in the shape of ill health or emotional upset, and a maintaining cause, which may be the continuation of the exciting cause but is at least as likely to consist of habitual misuse – habits of strain, for example, particularly those associated with wearing glasses.

DR BACH AND THE FLOWER REMEDIES

Dr Edward Bach (1880–1936), an English contemporary of Dr Bates, taught that all disease originated in the mind from negative emotions. After a lifetime's research in every avenue of healing science, including homoeopathy, to which he made great contributions, he found that in wandering the countryside he was intuitively drawn to certain plants that he associated with particular emotions. Later, more dramatically, he began to experience strange and unpleasant emotions out of the blue, which made him search for the plants whose essences would relieve them. When the remedies reached 38 in number these experiences ceased, and he concluded that his work was complete.

The 38 remedies relate to carefully delineated emotional states and, when sensitively used, are extremely powerful healers. A composite remedy, the 'rescue remedy', is valuable in every kind of emergency and trauma. A great advantage of the flower remedies is that anyone can begin to use them effectively with minimal training, whereas competence in homoeopathic prescribing, except for simple first aid, requires a long and intensive training.

Prescribing the flower remedies in itself encourages the development of insight into emotional states, enabling some people to develop great sensitivity and wisdom.

Dr Bach's point of view was unequivocally religious. He maintained that the power of the remedies was a gift from God, and that their effectiveness depended on the love and healing intent with which they were used.

Dr Bates recognised that negative emotion was a primary cause of poor sight; conversely we can recognise that failing sight is the first symptom of emotional dis-ease which will have more serious consequences if ignored and unchecked. Dr Bach's remedies afford a practical way of using this insight. By addressing the underlying emotional problem, the sight will be improved; by recognising the true meaning of poor sight, one can use it as a guiding symptom to help heal disease on every level.

BRAIN INTEGRATION

It has been commonly held for some time that there is a degree of specialisation of function between the two hemispheres of the brain. Many techniques refer to the importance of the relationship between 'left' and 'right' brain.

The 'left side' is normally associated with the hard, masculine qualities of structure and logic, embodied by the yang principle in Chinese philosophy and by the characters of Mars, Saturn and Uranus in astrology; while the 'right side' is identified with the yin, or feminine principle, also ascribed astrologically to the planets Venus, Jupiter and Neptune.

Some attempts to popularise the idea appear to reduce it to the dogma 'left brain bad, right brain good' which is a little simplistic to say the least. The esoteric disciplines, in describing these polarities in their various ways all stress the need for balance and integration – this is clearly displayed in the ancient symbol of yin/yang in which the black and white are inextricably interwoven, and in the mathematical symbol for infinity, colloquially known as

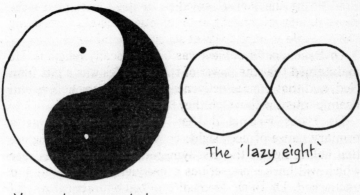

The 'lazy eight'.

Yin and yang symbol.

the 'lazy eight' which has been adopted to illustrate the constant flow and interchange between the two sides.

The idea that certain activities are exclusively 'right' or 'left' sided is obviously quite wrong. Such pursuits as painting, music and mathematics not only require a high level of integration to learn and perform successfully, it is also found that their successful and relaxed practice enhances integrated functioning – if they appear to make a demand which is one sided, that expresses a problem for the learner rather than a truth about the subject.

Muscle testing

The most reliable way of investigating the relationship of polarities in the human system appears to be through the various techniques of kinesiology, or muscle testing, which uses the activity of muscles to chart electrical potentials in the body and hence the activity of the brain. In this way one discovers that polarity patterns are very individual: the 'normal' functions of left and right hemispheres may be reversed (transposed hemispheres) and the dominance in eye, ear, hand and foot can show any permutation. It also appears that if communication between the two sides is impaired (midline block), normal function is emulated rather strenuously and inadequately by 'switching' –

rapidly alternating between the two sides instead of using them together.

Implications for vision

In applying these ideas to visual difficulties, the most obvious place to start is with the conditions involving definite imbalance, whether of the motor functions (as in squint), of the focusing ability (anisometropia), or of the 'signal strength' (suppression). More subtly perhaps, we can also consider the all-important relationship between the central attention and the peripheral awareness, and its physical equivalent in the relationships between the macula and the body of the retina and that between cone cell and rod cell vision generally, as aspects of the left/right paradigm.

Dr Bates was very clear that the central/peripheral relationship was crucial to the normal operation of sight, and this newer work makes it easier for us to understand, not only how right he was, but also why. It is also clear from experience, and entirely borne out by muscle tests, that improvement in all these and many other conditions is helped by relaxation and hindered by any kind of strain or effort. Apparently, the mental strain referred to by Dr Bates as the root of all visual evil, causes a tendency for the brain function to polarise whereas integration is aided by relaxation. Every new discovery in this field serves to underline just how far ahead of his time Dr Bates was in his thinking and further emphasises the importance of not suppressing visual symptoms but reading them for what lies behind.

4
THINKING ABOUT THE EYES – A HOLISTIC APPROACH

With the insights gained from the sources described in the previous chapter, among others, we can begin to develop an understanding by modelling the seeing process. An anatomical approach tries to identify the precise function of each component in order to deduce what it can do: our approach is to look at the operational requirements of the whole, as a computer systems analyst would do, and then try to work out how they can best be met.

WHAT DO THE EYES DO?

Most textbooks refer to the eye as the organ of vision, but it is more helpful and accurate to use Huxley's expression, 'organ of light'. The eye has many functions, all of which concern the processing of light, or of energy of similar frequencies. Seeing, although important, is only one aspect of this activity. Let us briefly consider some of the others.

Light refreshment
Sunlight is not only useful to see with, it is the essential element of life. The food that we eat, the fuel that we burn, the clothes that we wear are all composed primarily of stored sunlight. Light is also absorbed directly by the body as an essential ingredient in physiological processes. Light

absorbed through the eyes directly stimulates glands that regulate brain and body functions through hormonal secretions.

The attitude of medical science towards sunlight is rather ambivalent. Concern about the cancer- and cataract-causing properties of some ultraviolet rays is selling a lot of expensive sunglasses and making white skin universally fashionable. However, at the same time, people (the same people in many cases) are queuing up for full-spectrum light treatments to cure seasonal affective disorder (SAD) – the winter blues. In fact SAD is an interesting example of the time taken by medical science to catch up with common sense. For years those who complained of depression, lethargy and insomnia in the winter months were dismissed as hypochondriacs, while Dr Bates' advocacy of 'sunning' the eyes was derided as lunacy. But now it seems light is marketable. For indoor working (or domestic) environments, where artificial light is needed, full-spectrum (daylight equivalent) sources have great advantages, while spending time out of doors is also beneficial, and free; even an overcast sky yields as much full-spectrum light as any artificial source.

The window into the body

Normally light that enters the eye does not escape again. But with the aid of an ophthalmoscope it can be reflected out, and then the eye comes into its own as an inspection window. Through the ophthalmoscope one can observe physiological processes, such as circulation and even nervous function, which would otherwise be only partly revealed, even by invasive surgery. Ophthalmic diagnosis, however, should not be confined to eye disease; the condition of tissues within the eye can give valuable information on the bodily processes in general, always provided that the eyes are allowed to operate normally and that there are no purely local aggravations created by strain.

Iridology carries this idea forward. The iris, the coloured fibrous ring surrounding the pupil of the eye, is regarded as a complete instrument panel connected to every organ and function. The basic fibre pattern of the iris gives a useful indication of general constitution and the problems most likely to arise, while markings of individual segments can relate to problems in the corresponding parts of the body. The reliability of the procedure is controversial, but it is beyond doubt that the voluminous network of nerves that terminate in the iris fibres is quite superfluous to its limited physical function. The correlations between markings and organs proposed by iridology have been demonstrated in practice so many times that it can be at least as valuable as ordinary clinical diagnosis.

The mirror of the soul

If light does not ordinarily escape from the eye once it has passed through the pupil, that is not to say that the eyes cannot transmit their own energy and information. The expressive communicative aspect of the eyes goes deeper, and goes further back in time, than the use of atropine (belladonna) drops to create appealingly large pupils. The eyes display to the world every aspect of our feelings, including those we might prefer to hide – not for nothing are dark glasses the trademark of the dictator and the secret policeman. The connection between these responses of the eyes and our ability to see would make an interesting study in itself.

Interestingly, many people whose vision is really quite good will insist on wearing glasses, 'so as to see other people's eyes' whilst shielding their own. The enthusiasm for contact lenses is often ascribed to vanity, but it also often touches something deeper – an awareness of the need to communicate through the eyes with as little impediment as possible.

Eye-think

Dreaming is known to be an important activity for mental and physical health. It is a way of sorting and assimilating new impressions, without which we are liable to suffer from mental indigestion, and provides a pathway between the conscious and unconscious. Dreaming occurs during the rapid eye movement (REM) phase of sleep, when mental activity is mainly characterised by the so-called alpha waves, and this pattern is quite clear – no REMs, no dreams. This raises some interesting speculations: does dreaming operate like seeing in reverse, with the brain projecting pictures on to the retina? What would happen if the eyes were removed? What difference does it make if the eyes are unable to move freely?

It is because the functions of the eyes in seeing and in dreaming are fundamentally different that the practice of day-dreaming with the eyes open is generally frowned on by Bates teachers. When the eyes are open they should normally be properly directed for seeing: when they are closed they can do (within reason) what they like. Some meditative practices advocate an open-eye day-dreaming stare. When the vision is normal these practices, which have a specific purpose and are practised for a relatively short time, are probably harmless. But when priority is being given to improving the visual operation they are perhaps best avoided.

In the switchroom

Among the more intriguing recent discoveries concerning the eyes is that of eye modes, used in kinesiology and in neuro-linguistic programming (NLP). Directing the eyes in various ways turns out to be a way of channelling brain function in definite directions; used in this way the eyes act as switches to some of the brain circuits. We all use this unconsciously, for example in the case of deep sleep (characterised by delta and theta waves), in which the eyes will always be found turned up in their sockets. But this can be reversed; deliberately turning the eyes upwards, for example, is a sure-fire way of lowering the brain frequency.

Children tend to use memory and imaginative eye modes quite instinctively; a child who looks away when asked a question is not necessarily being evasive – she's probably thinking of the answer.

Implications

Taking into account all these extra-visual functions of the eye has important implications for the way we deal with the eyes in correcting vision.

- The use of glasses of any kind, dark glasses especially, cuts down the amount of light entering the eye, leading to what might be called optical malnutrition. Excessive sensitivity to light (photophobia) is therefore not a visual quirk, to be humoured with tinted glasses, but the optical equivalent of anorexia nervosa.

- If poor vision is due to strain, which disturbs the various muscle functions, this will additionally disturb the dreaming process and the mental 'switching' functions, as well as limiting the eyes' expressive capability – glasses that both fix and mask the eyes will not exactly help in any of these areas.

- Cases of squint and amblyopia (poor vision) involve the eye assuming unnatural positions: while a prismatic lens can neutralise the optical effect of misalignment, it will leave the position of the eye unaltered, or even fixed, with all that that implies. Similarly, forcible 'correction' by surgery will disguise the problem rather than cure it.

- Damage to the fibres of the iris, which commonly occurs in surgical operations, especially for cataract removal, will obviously rob the corresponding organs of this iridological monitor. The suggestion that the connection is reversible – that damage to the iris actually causes disease in the corresponding area – is unproven, but reasonable, and is supported by a number of anecdotes. The possibility should certainly not be excluded.

Consideration of all these points reinforces the argument for dealing with all visual problems, in the gentlest way possible, looking to restore harmony of function to the whole. A piecemeal approach – lens for this, surgery for that, drops for the other – is always likely to create as many problems as it solves.

VISUAL COORDINATION – A SYSTEMS APPROACH TO SEEING

And so what of the seeing process itself? In the light of Dr Bates' work and the other areas of study that we have mentioned, how do we make sense of it all?

Commonsense would suggest that the eyes should be so 'designed' that they could be 'calibrated' in use. Since physical growth depends on a number of uncontrolled variables, the idea that the accuracy of vision should be determined arbitrarily by the axial length, i.e. size of the eyeball, offends logic. Dr Bates' hypothesis, and the evidence he produced in confirmation, suggest that, in fact, any eye within a reasonable tolerance can be brought into effective coordination – as can, for example, arms and legs of various lengths and proportions. The following propositions develop some ideas on the nature of that coordination.

Feedback
• Seeing is a complex learned skill in which the mind controls the eyes through a sophisticated servo-feedback system.

In servo-feedback, information about the operation of a system is used to regulate the controls of that system; the simplest example is the governor on a steam engine, which monitors the running speed of the engine, automatically adjusting the steam pressure to keep it constant. Obviously, the more sources of information that are used and the more operations that are controlled, the more complex the process becomes.

The idea of vision depending on a learning process, as opposed to automatic development, may at first appear strange, but it agrees with all the known facts, as well as with common sense. It is universally agreed that sensing is an innate function of nerve cells, but that the interpretation of sensation has to be learned. The idea that the interpretation is fed back to control the direction and focusing of the eyes is likewise not at all controversial. The only area of doubt, then, concerns the extent of variability and the range of factors involved, and from Dr Bates' work we have learned that both are greater than generally supposed.

Considering vision in terms of coordination means it is more like than unlike an ordinary physical skill. Every parent has seen a baby mystified, then delighted, by the discovery of control over the hands, followed at length by the discovery that they are actually attached to the body; has seen the child crossly crawling backwards when it wants to go forwards, until eventually it submits to reality and does that which works; has heard the child's experiments in producing vocal sounds, which, gradually or suddenly, take on the shape of language. These are all complex coordinations learnt by a lengthy process of trial and error.

Before any of these childhood skills can be attempted, the process of learning to see will be well under way. The vacant wandering expression of a newborn only turns to a focused gaze once an enormous amount of information has been absorbed, countless experiments made and provisional conclusions reached as to what is the best way to go about looking at the world. The crucial task of the mind is to make sense of the world, and vision is useful in so far as it contributes to this. It follows that the skill of seeing must develop in parallel with knowledge of the world. It is impossible to achieve normal vision, even meaningless to speak of it, unless one knows quite a bit about what is being seen.

Memory and imagination

- Memory and imagination are employed in shaping the sensation of vision into a perception, which is in turn fed back as the basis of control of the eyes.

Every impression received is stored in memory. The impulse to make sense ensures that, very early on, a 'filing system' is set up in which the impressions are grouped and cross-indexed. Before long, every fresh incoming impression will be checked against a huge number of its predecessors to see where it will fit in. As the memory banks expand it becomes impractical to run every sensation through the whole lot, so each 'search' is limited to those fields most likely to be useful – we begin to form preconceptions. If a new impression fails to fit any known field, we request more information. This is the role of the imagination; the 'What is it?' of memory is projected into 'What might it be?' This leads to adjustment and movement of the eyes until a satisfactory answer is produced.

Without memory and imagination working in this way, not only would there be no perception, there would also be no control of the eyes. Instead of perception, vision would involve a meaningless jumble of chaotic instant impressions. Equally, the memory and imagination can only serve in this way where there is attention. As Dr Bates wrote, 'If the mind is not interested, the eye cannot see'. For a baby, interest in the environment is a fundamental condition of life, and its lack is a cause for serious concern. Many adults, however, regard it as normal, almost a

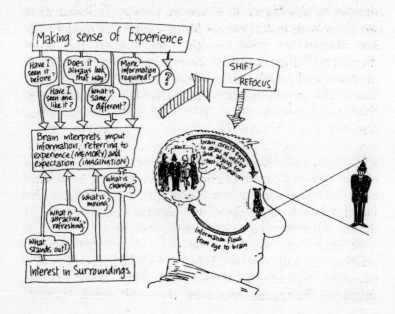

virtue, to lack interest and curiosity – and then they wonder why their eyes 'get bad'.

The other senses
- The visual process works best in alliance with the other senses, and suffers when isolated.

Because of the way we live, we tend to assume that vision is the primary sense. For a baby, however, this is not at all the case; the newborn lives much more in a world of touch, taste and smell. Although human babies' eyes are open from birth, it is clear that the visual impressions they receive take some time to become meaningful. A baby's first response to a new object is to hold it, taste it and smell it, and *then* to look for the visual correspondence to what has just been experienced at first hand. This runs precisely in parallel to the basic nature of sight, which is to identify objects at a distance, relating them to an immediate experience of things close to. In other words, sight functions as an extension of the primary senses, to extend the range of experience beyond arm's length.

How much the extended experience can mean will be limited by the degree to which we have assimilated what we know within that range. Many aspects of modern life are blamed for poor eyesight, one that is not often mentioned being the general corruption of sensuality. Lack of space, and consciousness of cost, makes 'Look but don't touch' the most important unwritten law of our society. Such injunctions as 'Keep off the grass', 'Don't pick the flowers', 'Don't handle the exhibits' are of course necessary, but damaging for all that. Smell and taste possibly suffer even more: our noses are faced with the alternatives of foul odours or synthetic air fresheners; food is deliberately standardised, to stimulate without surprising the jaded palates of those for whom eating is a chore or a social device, but rarely a simple relaxed pleasure.

Seeing, then, needs to be part of a total sensory relationship with the world, but it has for millenia had a secondary function as an extension, not of *sensing*, but of *language*. Language mediates the real world through symbols, and much of our seeing is concerned much more with symbolic information than with physical reality. This is not to say that books or, for that matter, computers are necessarily a bad thing, but I suggest that symbolic information is beneficial only to the extent that it improves or extends our contact with reality. To the extent that symbolic information reduces or seeks to replace our immediate experience, it is harmful, and the harm begins with the failure of the senses that are the very means of our contact with the world. Visual acuity is more or less measurable, but how do we measure touch sensitivity or compute its loss?

Vision develops as an extension of the primary senses, although very often it ends up being used entirely to process abstractions. On some level, then, if sight is to be restored, we must seek a better balance between the symbolic and the concrete aspects of seeing, and between vision in general and the primary senses.

Variability and certainty

• Normal vision is variable within certain limits. The variability reduces as experience creates relative certainty in the perception, and hence reliability of coordination.

Control of the eyes, the physical part of the ability to see, can only develop alongside its mental counterpart, the ability to turn sensation into perception. As we have seen, this involves, *inter alia*, the development of memory and imagination and the use of the other senses.

In many cases where there appear to be diagnosible motor problems, there is actually no fault in the system, merely insufficient information 'programmed' for it to run properly. There is no question of a baby's eyes refracting, tracking or converging accurately until it has had considerable experience, and even then the object needs to be familiar; many babies' 'squints', which are the source of great anxiety to parents, can be explained in this way. If the perception is not defined, the mechanism does not exist to cause the eyes to fixate in unison. As this mechanism develops, the eyes should normally come into alignment without outside intervention; if they do not, one should investigate the causes rather than interfere with the eyes.

There is currently a fashion for putting glasses on very young babies so that clearer optical information will supposedly better stimulate the visual centres of the brain. This attractive idea unfortunately assumes that the traffic is all one way; but from the point of view of the feedback operations it can only be catastrophically disruptive. This is not just a case of putting the cart before the horse, but of slaughtering the poor beast in order to fit an engine.

At the other extreme of life, elderly people are often prone to all the problems that come from their vision becoming excessively 'fixed'. Normal mature vision, most commonly (though not commonly enough) found in the age range 8–40, should be constantly variable, sometimes excellent (under ideal conditions or in relation to objects of special interest) and always within tolerable limits. It is helpful to be aware of these variations, while intolerance of change or of temporary variability is a major source of bad habits and strain. In the vision of children, for example, the greatest challenge comes from over-accelerated mental development. Both in education and in entertainment there is a constant pressure on children to be old beyond their years, leading to a mental sophistication that can overload the visual system and cause resentment if there is any apparent deficiency. Poor vision may then be seen as an escape, a way of cutting down the overstimulus. Glasses override this defence, institutionalising the split between perception and coordination as they increase the load. We have to accept that it is as reasonable for the visual system to require rest as for any other area of psychophysical activity.

Stress
- Vision will be disturbed by mental, emotional or physical stress. After short periods of stress it will return to normal, but if the stress becomes continuous, or if habits

of misuse are developed *in response to the experience of poor vision*, the feedback system will be prevented from working normally. Poor sight will then become the norm, with the eyes operating either chaotically or out of fixed habit.

Stress must here be understood in its broadest sense. Chemical toxins, even inappropriate food, can stress the human system, as can noise, lack of space, lack of freedom of choice, and a multitude of other things. This is not to say that everyone has to lead a perfectly serene, totally detoxified life, just that we should be aware of all possible angles.

A useful concept here is *appropriateness*. If I am happy, relaxed and interested in my surroundings, good sight is the appropriate response. If I am feeling sick, depressed, introverted or confused, the appropriate response will be defective vision – there is no reason why my sight should be normal when I feel so bad. When I cheer up and come back into the world, the conditions for good vision are restored; it *should* then come back to normal, although there are a number of possible reasons why it may not. If I spend a great deal of time being depressed and withdrawn, I may get so used to seeing a blur that I come to recognise that as normal. The coordination becomes permanently adjusted to this state and cannot alter it, even when it is clearly no longer appropriate. In a nutshell: I forget how to see. Alternatively, I may not forget entirely, but the co-ordination becomes uncertain; for example, I may snap out of a day-dream very quickly, 'leaving the eyes behind'. Left to themselves they would come back to normal soon enough, but I will not or cannot give them that chance; instead I begin to strain to try to force them to act. This straining can quickly become a habit, making a return to normal function impossible. Under the practical demands of life, many of us, from schoolchildren to clerks or executives, spend a great deal of time needing to see clearly under conditions of mental disturbance to which the appropriate response is a blur.

Permanent habits of strain, and the apparently inevi-

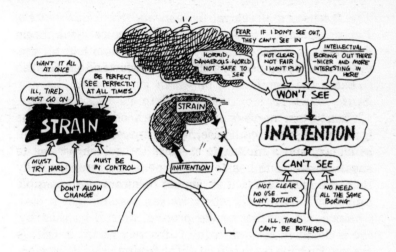

table 'need' for glasses, are the most likely, but not the only possible, outcome. Making the attempt to understand in what sense our poor sight is (or once was) appropriate for us is a useful step towards a situation where normal sight may be appropriate at all times. We have spoken of the usefulness of poor vision in indicating emotional disturbance, the first stage of dis-ease. Vision can only fulfil this function if it is acting freely and appropriately. If the eyes are operating out of fixed habits of misuse, they cannot respond in this way. Restoring connectedness between eyes and mind is not the same thing as improving the sight to normal, but it's an essential first step.

Central fixation
- The crucial factor in the normal operation of sight is central fixation, which depends on the constant stimulation by movement of the most sensitive part of the retina – the fovea centralis. When the vision is chronically disturbed, central fixation fails and this in itself causes further deterioration in acuity. A vicious circle develops, strain to see creating more blur, etc. This can only be remedied by making the restoration of central fixation a priority.

The mechanics of central fixation and the history of Dr Bates' discovery of its crucial importance have been described (see pages 8–12). One way or another, all the techniques developed by Dr Bates are focused on central fixation, the significance of which goes beyond the eye itself.

Clearly, any nervous structure such as a sense organ, feeding the brain with information, must have a complementary structure within the brain – a 'receiver', so to speak, tuned to the same frequency as the 'transmitter'. Since we can observe that central fixation is an essential aspect of the eye's operation, we can assume that it also figures in the parallel mental process; we can *see* that the eye is designed to work only in this way and it is fair to assume that the same is true of the brain.

Dr Bates went so far as to suggest that central fixation – the ability to give attention to one thing at a time within an integrated field of awareness – was an essential element of mental and physical health, and my feeling is that he was probably right. Here we are using the eye as a window, not just into the physiology of the body but into the very workings of the brain – and without using a scalpel or a microscope.

The use of glasses

- Corrective lenses never improve the vision; whether they stabilise it or cause further deterioration depends on individual factors. Since they encourage the eyes to adopt a habit of abnormal behaviour, while masking the true nature of the problem, they are as unwelcome as they are unnecessary and irrelevant.

If we are clear that visual disabilities are functional, and therefore alterable, and that they arise primarily from states of mind, there is no reason or excuse for prescribing glasses. To the extent that the poor vision is appropriate, it can be used as a reliable guide to the underlying problem; if it is inappropriate, i.e. if it stems from habitual misuse of the eyes, it can be remedied by visual re-education.

Giving glasses at the onset of a problem can only turn a

temporary aberration into a permanent habit since, in order to see through them, the eyes must constantly behave as they did when the glasses were fitted. It is noticeable that when glasses have been used for any length of time, the vision becomes less variable and the central fixation less defined. This is not surprising, since the normal mechanisms are being bypassed; misbehaviour is rewarded, clear vision is handed up on a plate and the searching movements and focal adjustments of normal vision are of no advantage – even a nuisance.

Optical prescribing is based on obtaining fixed measurements, and the way that testing is carried out is designed to obtain a precise fixed value as far as possible. Opticians, who spend most of their lives dealing with faulty vision, usually regard a fixed condition of sight as normal, and will go to great lengths to encourage it. Once fitted with glasses, the majority of eyes will fulfil this expectation nicely, while the minority who do not can frequently expect to be not taken absolutely seriously.

From an understanding of visual function it is clear that, in compensating for the inaccurate focusing of the eyes, glasses drive the eyes further and further away from the possibility of their working normally. The exact outcome depends on the particular causes and susceptibilities at work in the patient; some people wear the same glasses for years, while others 'progress' by leaps and bounds. Where there is no strong underlying cause, and if the interest in seeing is boosted, as it may be, by having the world presented more clearly, the sight may end up operating more or less normally, simply making an 'allowance' for the glasses. The cases where lenses appear to stabilise or even improve the vision come into this category; if being presented with a relatively clear image reduces the strain to see, the vision will improve as the eyes (relatively) relax. However, it is possible to stop straining without putting on glasses and anyone who can improve their vision with lenses could do even better without them.

But in the 'progressive' cases, which go inexorably from

bad to worse, there is evidently a powerful causation at work that is in no way addressed by glasses. The emotional picture usually includes an unconscious element of not wanting to see, or at least an ambivalence towards seeing.

Thus the eyes are caught in a crossfire between a conscious desire for clear vision, which sends the patient back to the optician for ever stronger glasses, and an unconscious refusal of the clear vision, which worsens the sight as fast as the prescription is increased.

These latter cases may need work on many levels, especially if the problem has progressed a long way, since the vision may be very poor indeed and the eyes subject to pathological change. An important interim approach is to work on reconciling the emotional conflict – Bach flower remedies and left/right or kinesiological approaches may be needed – and to accept a compromise level of vision that is practically adequate but diffuse enough to relieve the emotional pressure. Whatever further measures are used to improve the sight, they will only succeed to the extent that they are not eye-centred but person-centred.

Diseases of the eyes
• Diseases of the eyes arise from the coincidence of chronic malfunction, and its accompanying strain, with a constitutional predisposition to disease in general.

Disturbance of vision, as we have seen, is in many cases an indicator of disease in general. When the eye itself becomes diseased to the extent of showing pathological change, it is not sensible to regard this as a peripheral event; it must be taken seriously as an indicator of deteriorated general health. From a homoeopathic point of view we can say generally that predisposition (chronic miasms active in the body) will determine what kind of disease we get; the presence or absence of exciting causes, whether we get them or not; and the presence or absence of maintaining causes, whether we get better.

The eye disease picture will always include:
• Disordered functioning of the eye, either from habit or present emotional causes.

- The state of mind – whether or not it affects the function of the eyes.
- The constitutional state of health. Homoeopathy speaks of miasms – inherited chronic disease states that undermine the health and predispose to particular disease patterns.

Although it is quite clear that the eyes of people with normal sight very rarely, if ever, become diseased, the connection between eye disease and poor sight has been obscured by the opticians' insistence that most refractive error is physiologically and functionally 'normal', i.e. acceptable, for certain eyes. This position is made easier by the fact that most eye disease occurs among the elderly, most of whom are presbyopic (see pages 70–72), one of the conditions regarded as 'normal' in this age group.

Progressive myopia, where the physiological abnormality and its connection with the severe pathological complications have to be admitted, is treated as an exception; but it is not exceptional, it is merely an extreme form of the common process. The realisation that habitual refractive (focusing) error indicates continuous malcoordination and strain on the eyes makes it obvious that the eyes, if continually stressed in this way, will become the natural targets for any disease process going.

It should also be noted, however, that although the disease process is most obvious in the eye, it is not confined to that organ. In the nature of the case, small events in the eye will announce themselves by large impairments of vision. Furthermore, the transparency of the eye makes small pathological changes easy to observe. But disease is always of the system in general, and the underlying state of health must be the priority in any treatment that is to have long-term success.

No one would object to surgery or drugs to control a genuine emergency, but neither should anyone forget that these approaches do not deal with the cause. Most sudden events, like earthquakes, are actually predictable enough if one looks for the signs. My preferred therapeutic approach in all disease cases is homoeopathy; others may opt for

Chinese medicine, dietary therapies or herbalism. Provided that whatever approach that is used is based on the whole – and it works – then fine. In all cases, whether or not surgery is used, the combination of this kind of treatment with visual re-education should lead to the best result.

It has sometimes been reported that this or that expert has warned against 'doing eye exercises as advocated by Dr Bates' if you suffer from certain kinds of disease, alleging that it would be harmful. Now it may be that, in trying to learn from books, perhaps failing to understand the principles of relaxation and being generally over-eager, some have created strain instead of relieving it. But that is hardly the fault of Dr Bates. The Bates method in its practical aspect is entirely concerned with exploring and encouraging the normal relaxed operation of the process of seeing and, whatever the condition, that can only do good.

The improvement of vision
- The improvement of vision requires the elimination of influences causing or maintaining poor sight, including those of emotional distress, ill health and the wearing of glasses; and the re-education into proper habits of seeing, especially the normal relaxed use of eyes and

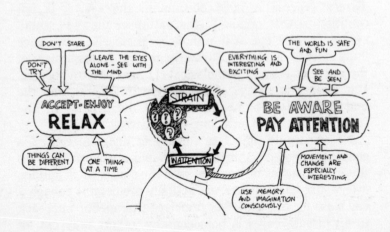

mind, and the re-establishment of the normal operation of central fixation.

A balanced approach is necessary. Simply discarding glasses will not by itself alter habits of seeing, and may make matters worse unless one also learns about visual relaxation. Learning proper habits of seeing is not at all the same as 'doing eye exercises'; the idea that one is to do some kind of optical circuit training to strengthen the eyes is utterly wrong, a complete misunderstanding of Dr Bates' work.

It is difficult, even dangerous, to try to learn practical skills from books (including this one) because we always tend to impose our own way of thinking on the words we read. Instead, we have to learn a different way of thinking, a process that may take a little time, for the simple reason that if our thinking were right we would have nothing to learn. F.M. Alexander put it rather well, as always: 'The right thing to do would be the last thing we should do, left to ourselves, because it would be the last thing we should think it would be the right thing to do.' His pupil, the great Alexander teacher Patrick Macdonald, perhaps put it even better: 'The trouble with words is that most people are

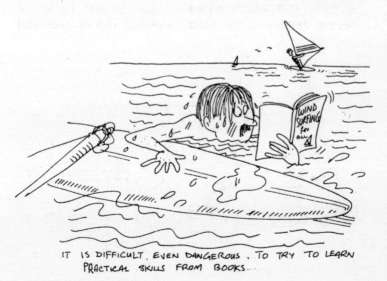

IT IS DIFFICULT, EVEN DANGEROUS, TO TRY TO LEARN PRACTICAL SKILLS FROM BOOKS...

more inclined to twist the meanings of words to fit in with the experiences with which they are familiar, than to accept new experiences in order to find out the meanings of words.'

That is why, in the Bates method, as in the Alexander Technique, the individual help of a teacher who has been through the process and fully understands the philosophical and practical difficulties is really essential; and why there is a great need for more such teachers, able to help their pupils accept new experiences of seeing.

5
THE CONDITIONS OF SIGHT

So far we have given a general account of the process of vision and the conditions under which it will deteriorate or improve. Poor sight takes many forms, according to the differing susceptibilities of individuals as well as to a variety of causes.

All practice starts from diagnosis, the identification and naming of the problem. Conventionally, each disease or abnormality is regarded as a separate entity, with a specific treatment aimed at ameliorating particular symptoms. Holistic thought seeks to trace all the manifestations of disharmony to their common cause.

The Greek myth of the hydra sums up the problem; cut off one head and two grow in its place. Somehow a way has to be found to strike to the heart. According to Dr Bates the heart of the hydra of poor sight is mental strain, and the purpose of studying, and initially differentiating, its various heads is to understand better their growth from this single cause.

Visual function and associated disorders are usually studied under five headings.

- *Motility.* This covers the movements of the eyes in relation both to a target and to each other. Motility problems have conventionally been approached in terms of muscle balance and nerve function, with treatment by surgery and drugs, correction by lenses and orthoptic exercises.
- *Refraction.* This includes all questions arising from the focusing of the eyes in relation to a target. Inaccuracies are conventionally described in terms of physical abnormality – the eyes being 'the wrong shape' for

51

normal vision – and treated mainly with glasses or contact lenses, although there is increasing interest in surgical techniques.

- *Perception.* The classification of a problem as perceptual normally takes it out of the field of the optician and into that of the visual psychologist, or even the neurosurgeon. The connection between perception and the physical aspects of vision is conventionally regarded as one-way; perceptual difficulties may arise from faulty refraction or motility, but the converse is not usually considered, since that would contradict the view that the motile and refractive errors have purely physical causes.

- *Pathology.* Since disease of the eyes are normally supposed to arise independently of other conditions, conventional treatments, where available, are always local, emphasising drugs and surgery.

- *(Dis)comfort.* The jargon for discomfort in and around the eyes, or caused by their use, is *asthenopia*. Where there is no pathology to account for the pain, the conventional approach focuses on uncorrected 'faults' of refraction or motility, and will attempt to relieve the problem by prescribing glasses. In cases where the vision is apparently normal, it may be maintained that there are latent problems, that the eyes only see 'normally' by straining – something that the glasses will relieve. When pain symptoms arise from the wearing of glasses, a sympathetic optician will juggle ever more complex prescriptions, while his less friendly colleague will pass on to another customer as quickly as possible.

In practice it is unusual for trouble to come singly. Even quite simple refractive errors often involve some degree of motile disorder, perceptual problems are inextricably bound up with the physical aspects of seeing, and, as we have seen, eyes that become diseased usually have a history of abnormal behaviour. Every case will reveal an individual profile, a different web woven from the common threads. With that caveat we can, nonetheless, discuss the more common conditions under their usual headings, always aware that the connections between events are more important than the distinctions.

MOTILITY DISORDERS

The normal movements of the eye are described as vergences, pursuits and saccades.

- Vergences are the movements by which both eyes are brought to bear on a common target.
- Pursuit movements are those involved in tracking a moving target, or a target seen from a moving position.
- Saccades are the small rapid movements involved in the maintenance of central fixation.

Vergent error

Vergent error may be symmetrical or asymmetrical. Simple symmetrical convergence errors – under- or over-convergence at a given distance – are a common cause of blurred or double vision, and of headache. It is commonly associated with refractive error; people with short sight often over-converge while people with long sight usually under-converge. In presbyopia inaccurate convergence is nearly always present, even when there is hardly any refractive error, and strain from this source may be the main culprit – see page 71. However, erratic convergence is quite easy to achieve, even with vision otherwise normal, especially after a few glasses of wine. It is usually simple to correct, and avoidance of strain and discomfort from this source will prevent the onset or worsening of other problems.

Asymmetric errors are usually called strabismus or squint. The usual picture is that, while one eye will fixate a target more or less accurately, the other will deviate in, out, up or down. One eye only may be involved, or the deviation may alternate between the two. Chronic strabismus usually involves refractive error in at least one eye, and perceptual problems can arise either from double vision or from the avoidance by suppression. The conventional treatment consists of surgery – advancing or 'tucking' a muscle to bring the eye into a cosmetically acceptable alignment – prismatic lenses to correct the remaining error, and orthoptic exercises that attempt to restore fusion. This approach is as wrong-headed as it is ineffective.

At one time squints were explained in terms of abnormalities of one or more muscles – they were too long/short or too weak/strong. Some doctors still talk in these terms, although most now accept that the problem is not with the muscle as such but with its innervation, i.e. with its nerve supply and stimulation. Despite this advance, muscle surgery is still widely regarded as a valid therapy.

We would go a stage further back, however, and suggest that, where there is faulty innervation of a muscle, we should really be concerned with the source of stimulus – the brain – and that, although physiology and mechanics do contribute to understanding, the main approach should be through education and coordination.

The truth of this is exemplified by three particular conditions. In amblyopia the relationship between the eyes constantly varies – one eye literally wanders around. It is usually associated with very poor vision in the affected eye, owing to lack of fixation, and more or less total suppression of the central vision.

Intermittent squints can appear in children of any age. The eyes will behave part of the time normally, squinting, apparently, as an emotional stress response or even a tool of emotional manipulation. Then there are the cases where a squint which has been 'successfully' corrected by surgery re-appears; I have seen cases in which two or three operations had made matters no better – worse, if anything. Clearly cutting the muscle had not removed the underlying problem – the hydra had merely grown two more heads. In all these cases there is every reason to suppose that the muscles are physiologically normal and doing as they are told. The question is, what instructions are they getting?

Parents of squint-eyed children are usually put under great pressure to have an operation performed as early as possible. The legitimising reason for this – that it will give the sight 'more time to develop normally' thereafter – is a convenient salve to the uneasy feeling that one is doing it mainly to be spared the sight of the disfigurement and the pitying looks of friends, neighbours and relatives. Everyone wants their child to be beautiful and perfect – that is nothing to be ashamed of – but, equally, a parent's real duty is always to the child's long-term interests.

Although not all children squint, there is no reason why they should not since, until some degree of fixation has been achieved, there is not basis upon which to sort out the coordination of the two eyes. Where a definite squint persists after fixation has clearly established itself there is cause for close attention, but not alarm and certainly not panic. If the squint is intermittent it is probably safe to ignore it; babies are sensitive beings, and constant poking, prodding and peering at them by all and sundry is as good a way to provoke a squint as any. If the squint is stable or alternating the first approach should be cranial oste- opathy, if only to eliminate mechanical problems such as might be caused by a difficult birth. If the birth was in any way traumatic, Rescue Remedy can be given as a 'consti- tutional' remedy at any stage of life. I am also very much in favour of routine homoeopathic treatment; young children have very little in the way of established habits and problems, and treatment on the dynamic level, which is what homoeopathy is, can have profound effects in the early stages of life.

If re-educational work is advised it should always be used sparingly and made into simple games. Some over- anxious parents think that a child will 'get on' better if subjected to a rigid daily exercise routine, instead of which it will become fretful and bored, thus defeating the object of the exercises. At the risk of being brutal, I must say that I find in this the same trait as in over-eagerness for surgery – wanting to do something for the benefit of one's own feelings rather than for the child's interests.

The great thing is to accept that there is plenty of time. The idea that a problem must be corrected by a certain critical date or the child's vision will never develop is absolute nonsense. As with all aspects of a child's development, one can encourage and steer it in certain directions but it will not stand being rammed into a mould.

So far we have spoken of squint as a developmental problem – a failure to establish normal coordination. Squints that appear later in life, after the sight has apparently developed normally, are nearly always of emotional origin. If I say that the highest incidence seems to occur in children whose parents have separated or where there is marital discord, it is not to pass any moral judgment, merely to point out that this unfortunate situation exemplifies a state of confusion, a division, a pull in two directions. A child of different susceptibility in a similar situation might react by becoming myopic or developing a number of non-visual problems in behaviour and health.

This is a book about eyesight, not marriage guidance, but a few principles are worth stating, for those who find themselves in this situation.

- A squint (or any other problem) that appears under these (or other stressful) circumstances is a sign of distress.
- It may also serve a covert purpose in causing the parents to focus their attention jointly on the child – or at least on his or her 'problem'. (The same may be said of behavioural 'problems'.)
- Submitting the child to glasses or surgery is victimising it for something that is not its fault. The visual disorder will do far less harm than such an act of scapegoating and betrayal.
- Children are resilient and adaptable. Don't waste energy feeling guilty about what you may or may not have done. Clean up the situation as well as you can, and create an environment with the most warmth and security possible, and the least ambiguity.
- Bach flower remedies, as necessary, for all parties in the situation will help to ease grief and help adaptation in changing circumstances.

- Re-educational help will be most appropriate if the visual problem does not resolve spontaneously after the resolution of the situation and return of emotional stability.

For some children, working on the vision with a friendly teacher may be a welcome distraction and source of therapy: others will experience it either as yet more victimisation, in which case it should be dropped, or as an opportunity for manipulating the parties, in which case great care, insight and, above all, honesty are required all round.

The keynote of squint in all its aspects is dissociation – the physical separation of the eyes, the rivalry, often leading to complete suppression of one side, and a difference in the visual acuity between the eyes (anisometropia). Our approach therefore reinforces Dr Bates' methods of relaxation and directed observation with modern brain integration techniques. Chapter 8 describes in some detail techniques for analysing and working with the practical side of cases involving squint.

Heterophoria is jargon for what might be called a latent squint. The eyes converge normally on a target so long as both can see it, but if one is screened from the target it will deviate relative to the other, which maintains fixation. According to many eye doctors this proves that it is not 'naturally' straight, or only straight under duress. They will argue for prescribing a prismatic lens, as though the eye were squinting in order to relieve strain, which they believe will otherwise cause harm.

There may indeed be strain involved with heterophoria, but if so it can be relieved by relaxation. In fact there seems no very good reason why the eyes should maintain vergence when only one can see the fixation point, except perhaps out of force of habit. Unless, therefore, there are concomitant symptoms of strain or visual difficulty, such a diagnosis is useful only as a possible predictor of dissociation under stress.

Pursuit errors

Pursuit errors are less common than vergent errors, but can be a real problem. Nystagmus is the condition in which the eyes flick from side to side in a conspicuous movement, unrelated to the normal seeing process; its opposite would be oculomotor paralysis, with the eyes unable to move at all. While true nystagmus is quite rare, there are plenty of people whose eyes do not track accurately – who, for example, cannot follow a bird in flight or who continually lose their place while reading. I have worked with several pupils who have had great difficulty with reading in that way, although their vision was otherwise excellent and there was no hint of anything that might be called dyslexia.

There are no conventional treatments for any of these states. If the vision is sufficiently disrupted, sufferers may be described as 'partially sighted' even though they see quite well for most purposes. They involve a loss of central fixation and a demonstrable strain, and are benefited by relaxation and re-educational measures.

Disruption of saccadic movement

Disruption of saccadic movement is an early indicator of strain and loss of central fixation. It is not likely to appear as a complaint in its own right, since most people are conscious neither of the saccadic movement itself nor of its loss, but it will be found as an element in most cases of any visual complaint. Working with conscious awareness of this movement (although many authorities say it is imperceptible, in fact anyone with more or less normal vision can pick it up) is an important means to improvement in a wide range of conditions.

ERRORS OF REFRACTION

Refractive error – the failure of the eye to focus accurately on a target – is the most common source of chronic poor vision. All refractive errors produce a degree of blurring, with or without accompanying sensations of strain, while astigmatism can also cause distortions of shape or multiple images in various configurations. These should not be confused with the binocular double vision caused by vergent error.

For centuries it has been assumed that the condition of the eye could not be altered, and that glasses were the only answer. The only problems were technological – getting glasses to work adequately in all circumstances. By the time of Helmholtz this point of view had been totally assimilated, and his *Treatise* is filled with laboriously compiled and calculated details of these incurable anomalies.

The refraction – the focusing ability – of the eye depends on a number of factors, amongst which are:

- The axial length of the eyeball, i.e. the distance from the front to the back of the eye.
- The total refractive index of the materials within the eye along that axis, i.e. the amount that these materials will bend the incoming light.
- In both the cornea (the clear area at the front of the eyeball through which the light enters) and the lens, the effects of curvature have to be taken into account. Indeed, recent work suggests that, far from being a uniform homogeneous structure, the lens in fact has an onion-like structure, consisting as it were of many lenses compacted together.
- Flexion of the lens, as well as alterations in the overall shape of the eyeball, will displace the fluid within the eye through which the light has to pass and by which the light is bent.

All in all there are far too many variables to make the impressive calculations found within the optical textbooks anything more than informed guesses.

In earlier chapters we have seen how Dr Bates discovered the basic variability of vision and what he and others have made of that discovery. In the light of our general discussion of the development of vision and the circumstances under which it deteriorates or improves, we can consider how the different conditions may arise in practice.

The flattening of the eyeball in hypermetropia (long sight) and the lengthening involved in myopia (short sight) are conventionally described as congenital structural anomalies, as randomly determined and unalterable as the length of our arms and legs. The only problem is that a slight difference in the length of a bone makes no difference to the usefulness of a limb, whereas in eyesight very small differences can produce the abnormalities of long- and short-sightedness.

According to the conventional teaching, these abnormalities of vision are physiologically and functionally 'normal', i.e. what one would expect for the eyes involved, and patients with these problems are routinely reassured that they are quite healthy. The cases in which this point of view cannot be sustained have therefore to be described as exceptions, or entirely different conditions. Dr Bates, on the other hand, maintained that most eyes are inherently normal and that refractive errors arise due to strain to see, the type of strain varying with the complaint. Thus he considered that long sight arose from a habitual strain to see at the near point, short sight from strain to see at a distance. He also noticed correspondences between the strain patterns involved in different complaints and the mental and emotional characteristics of the patients.

The first step in diagnosis is therefore to establish whether there is in fact a problem. It is well known that something like half the medical treatment given is for diseases that are iatrogenic, i.e. caused by medical treatment itself. More subtly, diagnostic procedures trend to create cases, either by inducing the patient to produce symptoms, or simply by labelling as a problem something that is perfectly normal and needs no intervention.

In optical physics it is well established that the behaviour of light itself is altered by the presence of an observer. In optometrics the stubborn belief that there is a true fixed condition of the sight, which simply has to be measured and corrected as necessary, ensures that many children are made to wear glasses who never need them.

Long sight in infants

It is often stated that babies are normally long-sighted. This apparently clear-cut observation conceals very questionable assumptions. It assumes that the refraction of the eye is significant, even though the child will have no firm conception of much that it sees. It also assumes (following Donders and Helmholtz) that the eye, when at rest, 'should' be perfectly emmetropic, i.e. accurately focused for distances from six metres to infinity. Observation apart, this is illogical. In designing and building any instrument, optical, musical or electrical, we would always make provision for calibration or tuning, which means always allowing a range greater than that required for normal operation – a margin of error. This ability to adjust in use extends the usefulness and insures against a variety of accidents. Similarly, the eye maintains focus by constantly refocusing a little in front of and a little beyond the target – as one would tune a radio. This would not work if the range of travel were limited to perfect focus for infinity; the focusing must be able to go at least a little beyond.

The likeliest explanation for these long-sighted infants, therefore, is that when the eye is perfectly at rest it will focus not at infinity but beyond; accurate focusing into infinity comes as the coordination is learnt, and the 'long sight' is a normal stage in the learning process. This question is currently of practical importance due to the fashion for putting glasses on tiny children in an attempt to speed up their visual development and enhance their learning ability. Like all the views questioned here (and by Dr Bates), this fails to recognise that the seeing–learning process is essentially circular and that any artificial interference is likely to be detrimental.

Long and short sight in children and younger adults

As to poor sight acquired after infancy, long sight is commonly ascribed to failure to grow, short sight to growing too much. This is supported by the numbers of long-sighted children diagnosed in early life and the steady increase in short sight as children get older. Since in the majority of cases the treatment (glasses) 'ensures' the correctness of the diagnosis (by creating the habit to fit), the statistics are neither surprising nor meaningful. In fact, either form of error can be acquired at almost any age, including the 20s and 30s when neither growth nor aging plays any significant part.

Dr Bates pointed out that sight testing is, for most people, a disturbing experience. Since mental disturbance adversely affects the sight, most people will therefore test below their normal level of vision. In one school he found that 50 per cent of children failed an eyesight test, but all passed at a second attempt, having familiarised themselves with the situation.

It is common experience in my practice to find a child, at first unable to read the largest letter on a test card (acuity less than 6/60), improve to 6/6 (standard vision), 6/4 (excellent) and beyond once they relax and are shown how to stop straining. Even with adults, nervousness and anxiety to please, to get the right answers, have to be put aside (a long job for some people) before the responses will bear any relation to their normal state of sight, and even then it will continue to vary. I would estimate that fewer than half the children given glasses for long and short sight actually need them in any meaningful sense, and that most of the remainder could avoid the need with very little trouble. In cases where a lot of work may be involved, glasses can be a pragmatic option, though never the ideal solution.

Leaving aside those whose visual problems are mainly diagnostic fictions, what of those who do have genuine difficulty seeing? As we have said, disturbed vision mainly reflects mental and emotional disturbance. I do not mean to imply that anyone wearing glasses is mad or in need of extended analytical therapy (although that may apply in a few cases); even quite small accidents can influence the development of a habit, and habits of thought, as Dr Bates wrote, largely determine how we see.

In the homoeopathic expression, an emotional upheaval may be the *exciting* cause of visual disturbance, but we have to look for the *maintaining* cause. If it is a continuation of emotional distress it will need healing. If (as is far more common) the poor sight is maintained solely by force of habit) – misuse – it is habit that must be challenged and altered; the original event may be of no relevance at all. At the same time, the challenge to habit may well throw up new emotional difficulties, hinging on resistance to change in the *status quo*, and these would certainly need to be worked through.

Generally speaking, the closer to the onset of a problem one begins work the less resistance there is from habit, although if there is a present emotional cause one may be in for an interesting time. With children it is best to start before glasses are given. After a few years getting used to 'specs' and adapting the personality, reversing the process may be quite traumatic. I am personally very wary of situations where most of the enthusiasm seems to come from the parents; but if the child is clearly very well motivated to get rid of their glasses, that is another matter.

Children appear to acquire poor sight – short sight especially – most commonly at certain critical ages. The biggest 'hump' is around puberty at 11–13, others being found at 7–8 and again at 15–16. This has been used to support the 'natural growth' theory, but lends itself equally to other lines of argument. One has to remember that childhood is a time of intense turmoil. I was once rendered speechless by a well-meaning mother saying 'Oh, but she's perfectly happy. I mean, children don't have anything to worry about, do they?' She had obviously completely erased the memory of her own childhood, and regarded her own child rather two-dimensionally. Even the happiest and best adjusted children in the most loving families can find life an enormous mystery, full of anxiety, confusion and unpleasant surprises – and most families fall just a little short of the ideal.

Puberty is the time when most of these pressures come to a head.

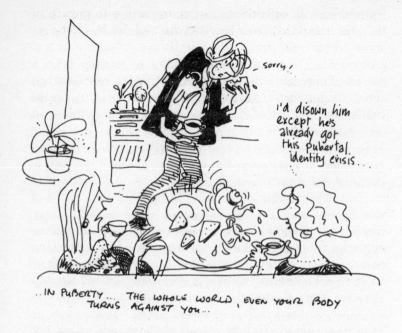

- The hormonal changes in the body play havoc with the emotions, provoking crises of identity and the need to re-evaluate social and family relationships.
- At the same time, life in most families involves an increase in responsibilities ('You're old enough to ...'), to say nothing of academic pressures, intensified for many by changes of school.
- Rapid physical growth disrupts coordination; dropping things, tripping over things and knocking things over become the norm. The whole world – even your own body – turns against you.

This entire scenario could be expressly designed to disrupt eyesight. Normal sight is a coordinated skill that works best when there is emotional balance and a healthy sense of connectedness to the outside world. Hormones playing ping-pong with the emotions, brooding introspection and a sense of isolation from the world do not help. Physical growth involves the eyes, but it does not follow that this will merely activate the 'time bomb' of latent short sight.

Rather, just as with the limbs, changes due to growth of the eyes mean that their new coordinated use has to be re-learnt. This re-learning goes on all the time that one is growing, but the extra rapid spurts of growth pose a special challenge and vision, like physical coordination, can be significantly disrupted. However, in many cases vision, like the use of the arms and legs, will stabilise in time without intervention.

The difficulty is that introspection and emotional instability are not helpful to this process, so that it becomes slower and less certain than it might otherwise be. At the same time, academic life makes its demands of reading and writing, both of which require a degree of clear vision. So, instead of being allowed to sort itself out peace-fully, the situation is likely to be aggravated by increasing anxiety about seeing, complicated by the development of all sorts of bad habits, until it is eventually settled forcibly by the ministrations of the optician.

Some will simply refuse to wear glasses at this age, or wear them for a time, then discard them, and come out perfectly all right. Many others will get into a considerable fix – unhappy in glasses yet unable to break out of the spiral of strain and poor sight. Yet others will accept the glasses as necessary, but at the cost of a shattering blow to self-esteem – feeling intuitively that they have failed in some way, or are being punished for who they are. I suspect that the extraordinary hostility exhibited by some wearers of glasses to the whole idea of natural vision improvement shows how hard they have had to work to bury painful (and quite unnecessary) feelings of revulsion and inadequacy in order to persuade themselves that wearing glasses is normal and that they are all right to be doing so. Having made such an investment, they are not lightly going to give it up, and anything that threatens to bring up those buried feelings is viewed as a personal assault.

Opticians and well-meaning parents try to sugar the pill with contact lenses, flattering fashionable frames and tinted glass for spectacles. The alternative is to validate the feeling against glasses; to let the young person know that they are right to dislike the idea of spending the rest of their life behind windows, and that, instead of 'stuffing' – internalising these feelings and accepting defeat – they can act on them and change the situation.

Because of this degree of emotional intensity and confusion, early adolescents can be quite difficult to work with on natural vision improvement. The most intelligent are more likely to succeed because they are able to detach themselves a little from their emotions, but there are always cases that are best left alone until they are ready, even if it means them spending a few years in glasses.

The slightly younger and older groups are on the whole easier, although indicated causes contain a good mix of confused coordination coupled with academic and social/emotional pressures. At age seven-plus, the sight has usually reached initial stability, but the child is taking up a slightly different place in the world; school turns from fun into more serious work, and so on. Again, in the teens, school exams have a way of coinciding with important social adjustments, and the same pattern is carried on through further education, starting work, professional exams, career changes and the rest. All of these events may give rise to temporary disturbance of the sight that will either normalise with suitable encouragement or become permanent through anxiety, strain or the use of glasses.

The events described are of course the routine stuff of many lives. More extreme situations, giving rise to more vivid symptoms, require great caution in deciding how, or whether, to proceed. Everyone's life has emotional ups and downs, but not everyone's vision is affected – not all have the same susceptibility. Emotional turmoil will always find its outlet, in dreams, in behaviour, in skin complaints, or worse. That is why it is no good trying to *make* the eyes work; one has to understand and remove the cause of the trouble.

In the same way, difference of susceptibility, rather than physical difference in the eyes, will distinguish long sight from short, and this is commonly revealed in the make-up of the personality. Both conditions display a lack of connectedness to the world as it is. Short-sighted people tend to want to leave the world alone (and hope to be left alone themselves), while long-sighted people tend to find the world not as it should be (and try to put it to rights). We can characterise the long-sighted personality as more concerned with other people's business than his own, given to generalising, hating to be bogged down in details, unable to see what is under his nose. In contrast, the shortsighted personality wants to let the world go by, has his head in the clouds, can't see the wood for the trees, can't see past the end of his nose. These are obviously gross caricatures; however, they do contain the odd grain of truth. Some individuals display the types very clearly, others show just a few hints within generally well balanced personalities, but there is enough to it to make guessing someone's spectacle prescription on the basis of 15 minutes' conversation an interesting variation on the game of guessing their sign of the zodiac.

It has always been generally assumed that the sight dictates the personality; myopes (people with short sight) have been supposedly inclined to books and studying, while those with long sight (hypermetropes) have been disinclined to these activities because of their vision. The converse is in fact equally likely, but it probably comes nearest to the truth to say that sight and personality grow together, woven out of the same stuff.

This raises the question as to whether, in attempting to normalise the sight, we are in some way denying individuality and trying to make everyone alike. Definitely not. The essence of individuality is to have options, and to be able to choose between them. The point about chronic poor sight is that it is stuck in a rut of fixed habit – not much individuality there. Also, to allow the sight to function normally implies that we will also be comfortable with its idiosyncracies, so that in fact it will express individuality more fully. The goal is to restore connectedness, to let the sight respond appropriately to what is happening and what is needed as much of the time as possible. I call in evidence the psychiatrist and analytical psychotherapist M. Scott Peck, who has defined mental health as 'a process of dedication to reality at all costs'. That is a valuable thought to apply to eyesight, in terms both of internal reality – the integrity of our coordination – and the truthfulness of our response to external reality, to the world out there, which includes optical accuracy, but much more besides. The greatest mistake we could make is to confuse the 'sum of our bad habits with the totality of ourselves'.

Astigmatism

Astigmatism has acquired a curious mystique due to confusion about its nature. Ironically, this is in a way appropriate since confusion is the key characteristic of astigmatism, but it need not be as confusing as all that.

Whereas in 'ordinary' long and short sight the eye refracts all light rays with the same degree of error, in astigmatism the error varies in different planes. This gives rise to a variety of visual effects: most commonly there will be a difference in the degree of blurring of parallel lines or stripes according to whether they are viewed vertically, horizontally or at some other angle; there may also be definite distortion of shapes – circles may appear oval, or segmented for instance.

In optical prescribing, straightforward long and short sight are corrected by lenses formed as sections of a spherical surface. The smaller the radius the stronger the lens (think of a small circle cut from a football for a fairly weak lens or from a tennis ball for a stronger one). Astigmatism is corrected by introducing an element of 'cylinder' (think of a section cut from a tube), the combination of spherical and cylindrical elements forming a complex curved shape somewhat like a section of a rugby ball. To make this work the prescriber needs to define the axes of the refractive error – two lines at right angles to each other which indicate the greatest and least degrees of the error – and ensure that the lens is worn in exactly the right position.

Thus an optician's prescription which reads:

R: SPH −2.5 CYL −0.25 AX 76

is specifying a basic correction (for short sight)of 2.5d with additional correction of 0.25d at an angle of 76° to the reference plane.

Because the technique of calculating and grinding these odd-shaped lenses was first developed in England, astigmatism was known for many years as 'the English disease' among more conservative continental opticians who were sceptical of the benefits of going to such lengths when good results could usually be achieved by ignoring small amounts of astigmatism and prescribing simple spherical lenses.

One of the most serious misconceptions that many people have about astigmatism is the idea that it is an actual disease. It is of course nothing of the kind – simply an error of vision which is not totally symmetrical. The word itself – 'a-stigma-tism' – means, simply, 'pointlessness' – there is no single clearly defined focal point. The conventional optical explanation and justification for aggressive prescribing is that the fault is inherent in the eyeball – either the cornea or the entire globe is supposed to be congenitally distorted.

Dr Bates found, however, that astigmatism could appear, disappear and change its form with great ease; in fact it is the most volatile and variable of all the visual disorders, reflecting a general lack of coordination and balance in the activity of the eye muscles rather than a particular fault in any one of them.

Prescribing lenses for small degrees of astigmatism definitely tends to create the problem it claims to solve and it can be argued, if one accepts Dr Bates' basic premises, that all astigmatic prescribing is likely to do far more harm than good. In the early stages of learning the Bates method, it is very common experience for astigmatism to change so frequently and drastically that there is simply no point in attempting to correct it. If glasses cannot be done away with immediately then the best solution is often to find a simple short- or long-sight prescription which gives adequate vision and comfort and sort it out from there.

All Bates teachers agree that working on the visual aspect of astigmatism without addressing the underlying mental condition is like collecting frogs in a bucket – entertaining, but ultimately frustrating and a waste of time. The keynote is always *confusion* – struggling to make sense, trying to do too many things at once. It is in that sense the condition of the times we live in – overcoming it has a lot to do with the relief of nervous strain, the achievement of tranquility and the development of a clear sense of purpose. More than any other condition, astigmatism demonstrates that clearly focusing eyes need the direction of a clearly focused mind.

Refractive imbalance – anisometropia

Some people have identical vision in both eyes, others show considerable differences. Difference in acuity due to refractive behaviour is jargonised as *an-iso-metropia* (not-the same-focusing). It may or may not co-exist with a motility problem such as squint and/or complete or partial suppression of one eye; there may also be a degree of 'specialisation' – a preference for using one eye for distance, the other for close work. Within limits aniso-metropia may be tolerable, even normal, but it commonly indicates imbalance in the eye–brain connections.

The common expression 'lazy eye' is misleading. The retarded eye is usually not so much lazy as suffering under considerable strain. It does not need to be 'made to work' but allowed to function properly and integrate with its partner through relaxation.

Accommodation errors

Here we have:
- *Presbyopia*, alias *pseudohyperopia*, alias old age sight, and ...
- *Accommodative spasm*, or, if you will, *pseudomyopia*.

And that's quite enough in the way of long names.

Like true long and short sight, these two conditions can

be considered as two sides of the same coin. In presbyopia there is difficulty in accommodating to the near point, although distant vision may be normal. In accommodative spasm the difficulty is with distance, while near vision is much better than in true myopia. The traditional explanations for these conditions focus on the lens and the ciliary muscle – the supposed agents of accommodation. Dr Bates, however, regarded them simply as varieties of aberration in the overall coordination. Both cases are characterised by an initial slowness in changing focus, compounded by strenuous attempts to speed it up that, in fact, have the opposite effect, causing the mechanism to 'seize up'.

We tend to assume that the eye is always automatically in focus on whatever we happen to look at. In fact, of course, the change of focus from one distance to another takes a certain time, which can be demonstrated and measured. The time lag is usually short enough to be imperceptible, maintaining the illusion that the change is instantaneous, but if the movement slows ever so slightly it will become noticeable. Once this happens impatience and irritation quickly lead to strain, at which point the eyes become stubborn – they do not like to be bullied.

Presbyopia often occurs together with under-convergence, or obvious discomfort in close convergence. In many cases I suspect the convergent error comes first, and that straining against it slows the change of focus. Either way, improving the convergence flexibility (it may take a long time to give up that effort) always makes it easier to sort out the focus problem. The fact that the two aspects are so closely related adds further support to Dr Bates' contention that both are functions of the external muscles.

Accommodative spasm, the reverse case, is probably most prevalent among those who read and write a great deal. Whereas presbyopia shows itself when one comes in from the garden and picks up a book or newspaper, only to find it blurred, accommodative spasm is revealed when looking up from the accounts to see the time and finding oneself unable to read the clock. Both conditions are easy to avoid and to remedy, especially in the early stages, if one is willing to slow down and *relax*.

Chaotic refraction

This is my name for a condition not generally described. Normal vision shows a balance of stability and variation – homoeostatic equilibrium in fact. The usual refractive errors are characterised by excessive stability – fixity instead of variability. In contrast chaotic refraction is characterised by excessive variation without stability; the eyes appear to change focus continually and randomly, disrupting the vision in a way that no lenses can correct. It is difficult to know how many such cases there may be, since those beyond the help of opticians tend to be categorised by the catch-all term 'partially sighted'. People who have great difficulty getting used to glasses or needing frequent changes may in fact be 'chaotics'. As usual, efforts to control the problem directly make it worse; an indirect relaxed approach, however, yields good results. This is a good example of a condition, albeit an unusual one, which appears to be more readily explained by Dr Bates' hypothesis than by the orthodox teaching.

Progressive myopia

I have placed progressive myopia last in this section because, although strictly a refractive problem, it borders on pathology and is in fact described in many places as a pathological problem.

Some people go a little myopic at some stage in their lives, then stabilise; others deteriorate over a period and then stabilise. But in progressive myopia the sight goes on and on deteriorating. Since this does not fit the standard theory of myopia, eye doctors have described progressive myopia as a distinct condition of unknown pathological origin. We would say, on the contrary, that it is an extreme and accelerated form of the syndrome found in many cases of 'standard' myopia – disconnection from visual reality and a vicious circle of strain, stronger lenses and worsening vision.

All refractive problems are likely to be excited by emotional causes and maintained by a variety of factors, including the wearing of glasses. To the extent that the original cause is removed or forgotten, and the problem is maintained through habit, the situation is likely to stabilise or deteriorate only slowly. To the extent that the original negative state of mind is still present, deterioration will be more rapid.

In progressive myopia the eyes are caught in a conflict between the conscious and unconscious. Consciously one wishes to see clearly, for its utilitarian benefits; unconsciously, for whatever reason, there is a refusal to see. Consciously, one goes to the optician for stronger lenses to overcome the problem with the eyes; unconsciously one shrinks from the clear vision they provide.

Progressive myopia is not the easiest condition to work with, for a number of reasons. Unaided vision may be so bad as to be intolerable; and even if it is actually quite reasonable, there is often a perverse insistence on using lenses 'to make things clear'. Contact lenses, especially, will be favoured as a way of denying the problem. But if there is to be improvement the issue cannot be evaded. Acknowledging the split between overt and covert intentions may be uncomfortable, unwelcome, even impossible, and if attempted may lead into areas beyond the teacher's competence; Bates method teachers are not trained as psychotherapists, and there are as yet few therapists to whom one might refer who share out understanding of the significance of vision.

The best approach I have found is to work with flower remedies and to explore the visual experience, seeking to accept stability of the vision, with lenses if necessary, at a compromise level – adequate, though less than perfect – refusing further increases in prescription. It must always be remembered that just leaving glasses off is nothing; the point is to learn to use the eyes without strain.

In very far advanced cases, return to normal unaided vision may not be possible, as the eye can be permanently distorted by the stresses involved. The first aim in such cases is always to prevent further deterioration, then to see what can be done. In an ideal world, proper preventive work at the right time would ensure that no one would get into such a state. Meanwhile, approaching the problem from a broad perspective offers the best chance of doing something useful.

PERCEPTION

Strictly speaking, all visual problems involve perceptual difficulty. It is faulty perception that maintains the squint or the short sight; any disease of the eye nerve or brain will disrupt the perceptual process; it is after all the linchpin of the entire visual operation. There are, however, certain problems, in so far as they can be disentangled, that belong under this heading rather than any other.

Suppression

The habit of seeing through one eye only is surprisingly widespread. The conventional explanation, that suppression arises in squints as a device to prevent the inconvenience of seeing double, sounds plausible up to a point. However, there are many cases of squint without suppression, the usual strategy to avoid double vision being to make the squint worse so that the images are more widely separated and one can be ignored. Equally there can be suppression without squint or any other problem. (One young man had perfect vision in both eyes and normal vergences but 'saw' entirely through one eye.) It is generally assumed that the eye with worse vision (if there is a choice) will be suppressed, but this is not necessarily the case. One boy had perfect vision in one eye and high myopia in the other; he could not see clearly unless the myopic eye was either corrected or covered.

When suppression, squint and anisometropia are combined it is helpful to think not of one as causing the others, but of both or all arising together, along with any other problem, from a common cause. The most productive approach to understanding and working with this problem is the brain integration model described earlier (see page 28). The conventional use of occlusion therapy (patching) – keeping the dominant eye covered for long periods – and of exercising with stereoscopes (devices for viewing pairs of images at the same time, one image for each eye, such that the images are combined to give a three-dimensional effect) can be reasonably effective; indeed, Dr Bates himself practised in this way for a time. But it is better to work rather more subtly to uncover, then overcome, the blocks to integration. There are practical techniques that may be used but it must always be remembered that the procedure is not mechanical – if it is to do any good, the process needs to be entertaining and relaxing.

Colour vision

Discussion and investigation of colour perception is fraught with difficulty. Whole books are devoted to techniques for standardising light sources and reflective surfaces in a way that will allow even the beginning of scientific evaluation. In all probability, no two people will have identical colour perception; nonetheless, most people manage to reach a consensus about the difference between blue and orange, for example, and those who are unable to share in that are at a disadvantage.

Since colour perception depends ultimately on the photochemical activity of the retinal cone cells, I had long assumed that the common forms of colour blindness were due to abnormalities in the pigment or nerve structure. This view was challenged when I had the opportunity to work with a colour-blind man who came to see me about something else. It transpired, in this case at least, that his colour blindness was worsened, if not entirely caused by, strain, and that the practices of resting the eyes and developing relaxed central fixation improved his colour perception enormously. This seemed to imply that the retinal cells, etc., were normal but that the process of perception was disrupted under conditions of strain. As with all visual conditions, the vicious circle would operate with increasingly anxious and strenuous attempts to distinguish colours, making matters steadily worse. Other reported cases show similar features, suggesting that, while the area of colour perception obviously needs further investigation, this fairly common problem is not at all incurable and may be quite easy to help in many cases.

Two-dimensional vision

A surprising number of people apparently see in a very two-dimensional way. Does this apply to you? If '3-D' films, or pictures viewed through a stereoscope seem 'more real than real', then very likely so.

Strictly speaking, we do not actually see solid objects, but only the images formed on the retina by light reflected from objects, and these images are essentially two-dimensional. Nonetheless it is possible, and extremely desirable, to experience the world as solid and three-dimensional. The way that the retinal pictures are rendered into this 'solid' experience is possibly the most mysterious aspect of the whole visual process: it is conventionally assumed that this is an automatic result of the fusion of pictures between the two eyes, but experience shows that there is rather more to it. Plenty of people have perfectly normal binocular vision but still see in a very flat way. (Equally, one can with a little practice develop an extremely good feel for space, distance and velocity through one eye, so although binocular fusion and 3-D vision are clearly related they are definitely not at all the same thing.)

Most people would not be aware of a deficiency in this respect unless they had the opportunity to compare it with something different. When that opportunity comes about it may be quite a surprise, as it was for me and for several of my pupils, to realise how much had been missing. How does this state of affairs come about?

In discussing the development of sight, I suggested that in the natural order of things eyesight is a secondary attribute, both in the sense that it is less important in the early stages of life and also in that it depends on the prior development of the other senses, especially touch, in order to become usable. In the same way, reading assumes prior development of the basic skill of seeing.

A great deal has been written over the centuries on the effects of reading on eyesight. What is not generally considered is that reading entails a completely different use of the eyes from the ordinary kind of seeing. Decoding signs and symbols whose meaning is entirely outside themselves is a very different activity to looking at a concrete object whose meaning is, so to speak, self-contained. The dependence of our culture on written information means that in many cases we act as though reading were the only worthwhile use of human vision, whereas it is a complex and problematic skill which has needed a lot of strenuous adaptation to acquire at a late stage in our evolution. Vision needs to be integrated with the other senses but reading mostly leaves the eyes in a kind of limbo, requiring the maintenance of clear focus, but not giving very much visual (as opposed to mental or emotional) stimulation. In short, it demands a great deal of the eyes while giving very little back.

Two kinds of difficulty come from this source: confining one's interest to information presented in a two-dimensional form creates a habit of looking at everything that way, while the simple fact that reading material is arranged on a plane surface goes against the eye's natural habit of constantly changing focus. As an experiment, try reading alternately from a smooth page and a crumpled one and see which looks clearer (it only works as long as the eyes keep moving). The answer to both difficulties is to find a sense of proportion: to allow direct experience of the world to regain its primacy so that reading can operate as part of that rather than as a substitute for it.

In the Bates training, great emphasis is laid on the experience of movement in spatial relationships and the correspondence between sight and touch. When these lessons are learned, reading can become a benefit rather than a burden to vision, and increase, instead of diminishing, our knowledge of the real world.

Reading difficulties – dyslexia

Reading is an awesomely complex undertaking that is too much taken for granted. Like all symbolic activity, written language offers the possibility of transcending our immediate experience, but needs to maintain contact with that experience to be of value. This is recognised in the practice, common in continental Europe, of deferring the study of reading and writing to the age of seven, using the kindergarten years to concentrate on developing sensory experience and motor skills. In the UK, for some reason, precocity in reading is regarded as a mark of an intelligent child and caring parents; the trend is to insist on starting at every younger ages, sanity in this respect being apparently confined to the Waldorf schools based on the precepts of Rudolf Steiner.

The world is not clearly divided into literate/illiterate, nor into dyslexic/'normal' readers. The ability to perform reading tasks varies widely, and individual abilities will vary at different times. Rather than thinking of dyslexia as a distinct condition, like measles, it is probably more helpful to think of it as a blanket term covering one end of

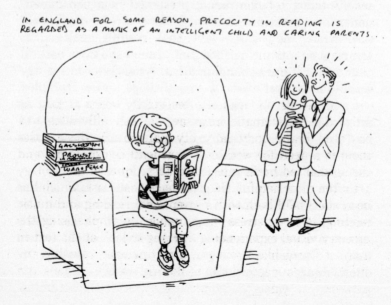

IN ENGLAND FOR SOME REASON, PRECOCITY IN READING IS REGARDED AS A MARK OF AN INTELLIGENT CHILD AND CARING PARENTS.

a broad spectrum of ease and difficulty in processing words. A degree of dyslexia can be induced in most people under some circumstances, as easily as a degree of myopia, and there is every reason to suppose that the development of an identifiable problem fits the common pattern of visual disorders. Either bad habits build up insidiously so that by the time the consequences are noticeable they are well ingrained as part of the 'normal' experience; or else a temporary difficulty (for example, as a result of fatigue or stress) evokes a straining response, making it permanent. Dyslexia is often thought of as a purely perceptual problem, but in many cases there is clear evidence that strain causes disordering of the eye movements in reading. Since these movements are effected through the extra-ocular muscles, disruption of this aspect of the coordination is as intelligible as those involving, say, squint or myopia, and can occur equally well in combination with such other problems, or alone.

Anything that breaks the vicious circle of strain and failure will be a great benefit, and with chronic 'failures' it is obviously preferable that a new technique should show results quickly, before another round of disenchantment and strain sets in. For that reason, short cuts like the polarising pink goggles, which have been introduced by some specialists in the field and which appear to work by simplifying the visual information, leading to success and relaxation, are to be welcomed.

Some kinds of dyslexia, especially those involving mirroring or systematic order reversal, generally relate to a confused brain–body laterality pattern. In these cases there is a need for work on the general coordination, and the specialised brain integration techniques of kinesiology are often most helpful. One approach that I use, which has been successful both with conventional reading and music reading, is to de-stress the situation by emphasising the primary visual experience – learning to look at the text in a relaxed way, like looking at a picture, and refusing any effort towards 'decoding' but allowing the connections and patterns to emerge. Simple exercises to 'programme' effective scanning patterns and conscious use of the central–peripheral relationship have been as helpful in this kind of difficulty as any other visual disorder.

Perceptual difficulties with glasses

Glasses, although they are intended to 'normalise' the vision, actually create a variety of perceptual problems.

For a start, they certainly add to the two-dimensional habit, literally presenting the world on a screen and virtually eliminating depth of field, while at the same time allowing the end of clear vision to be gained without employing the means-whereby of central fixation. They cause distortions, sometimes severe, in perception of size, distance and movement. Helmholtz, himself rather short-sighted, noted that when walking in the mountains, he felt surer of his footing, especially downhill, with his glasses off, though he would put them on to admire the view (an admirably pragmatic approach). Dr Bates also noted that glasses always dull the perception of colour, in turn reducing the definition of form, thus making the focus less certain, so requiring stronger glasses, and so on.

Where the eyes refract differently (anisometropia) the different kinds of lens may give a marked difference in image size (aniseikonia), creating problems in fusing the two images. This is especially prevalent where one eye has had its lens removed because of a cataract (aphakia). The best answer to all these problems is to stop using glasses and learn to see naturally. Even where this is not entirely feasible, the practice of relaxed attention will help co-ordination adapt to vision and, hopefully, improve vision at least enough to allow a complex prescription to be simplified, thus at least reducing the complications from that source.

6
DISEASES OF THE EYE

Strictly speaking, there is no such thing as an 'eye disease', the eyes show symptoms of general disease to which they are susceptible. This applies equally to conditions such as multiple sclerosis (MS) which have eye symptoms alongside others, as to the styes and inflammations which probably indicate blood disorders, and to the regular 'eye diseases'. Having said that, organic eye symptoms should always be thoroughly investigated by a physician or optometrist. Early diagnosis means that there is time to consider the broadest range of options.

Eye symptoms do us a favour in making us aware, very early, of slight chemical imbalances, but also irritate, making us want a 'quick fix' which is rarely in the long term interest. The orthodox treatments offer this quick fix, treating the symptoms in isolation with surgery and locally acting drugs. In an emergency there may be no choice, but in a chronic condition it may be worth considering alternatives. It is really the general disease that needs healing: whole person approaches such as homeopathy or Chinese medicine are required, together with appropriate attention to such questions as nutrition, elimination and exercise. It is important however to avoid anything that will add strain to the eyes, so avoid violent or strenuous movement and don't even *think* about the 'stretch and roll' style of eye exercises found in some books (not this one). In conditions which threaten blindness, *fear* can become the dominant factor; establishing emotional balance, through therapy or with the help of remedies, is always an essential step. The Bates method is not a treatment, but is often a valuable complement to the treatment of choice; whatever the condition, it can only be helped by methods that relax, reduce stress and improve co-ordination. Looking at visual stress is potentially a means to learn a lot about the general processes involved, as well as to keep the best possible vision.

Cataract

Cataract is the name given to any condition in which the lens of the eye loses transparency.

When cataract occurs congenitally in children it must be treated constitutionally, starting as early as possible and maintaining treatment as long as necessary. Visual re-education will be indicated to overcome any obstruction of visual development; even if temporary, the obscurity of the lens will interfere with the development of central fixation, with possible later complications.

In older people cataract occurs most commonly as a sequel to presbyopia ('old age sight'). Its development seems to be encouraged by inflexibility in the use of the eye, so the encouragement of relaxed and flexible action is most important. It can also arise very rapidly in response to emotional strain or shock, and this must be dealt with as necessary. There has always been an association between cataract and diabetes, and recent research has shed light on this connection. It appears that excess sugar in the bloodstream which cannot be properly metabolised forms complex (and opaque) compounds with body proteins, especially with the crystalline proteins of the lens. The ability to metabolise sugar reduces with age, and stress is known to affect the metabolism in general, so this work demonstrates a likely link between the various factors known to be involved.

The conventional treatment for cataract is to remove the entire lens surgically, either replacing it with a plastic implant or simply correcting the vision with spectacles, contact lenses, or a combination. For a number of reasons, including ease of removal and the risk involved, it is customary to allow the cataract to 'ripen' to the point where vision is almost lost before operating. That being so, cataract patients have nothing to lose and everything to gain from trying alternative approaches while they are waiting. If the alternative succeeds, surgery will be unnecessary; if not, it is still available.

Even in cases where surgery is ultimately necessary, learning the Bates method can do a deal of good. Allowing the cataract to obscure the eye as it ripens involves the risk of great strain and loss of central fixation, while the adjustment to seeing with the peculiar lenses used post-operatively involves great perceptual difficulties. Study and practice of the art of seeing will help avoid complications and ensure that the vision is as good as possible.

Glaucoma

Glaucoma is a condition of raised pressure in the eye. A fluid called the aqueous humour is constantly secreted into the front chamber of the eye (between the cornea and the lens). This fluid is then normally drained into the canal of Schlemm, a tubular ring around the margin of the cornea, which, like a land drain, ducts the aqueous fluid away.

If the secretion of aqueous humour is greater than the drainage, the intraocular pressure – the pressure within the eye – will obviously rise. Because the sclera, the envelope of the eyeball, is not elastic such excess pressure will be concentrated at the weakest point, which happens to be the optic disc, the entry point of the optic nerve (see diagram on page 84). Subjected to this excess pressure, the optic nerve begins to 'die' from strangulation, leading to progressive loss of vision. The outer fibres of the optic nerve, corresponding to the periphery of vision, die first so the effect is of a loss of visual field.

Onset may be sudden (acute glaucoma) or insidiously gradual (chronic glaucoma). Acute glaucoma is always a medical emergency, with the eye painfully inflamed and swollen, and rapid loss of vision, and in nearly all cases requires urgent surgery to save the sight. Chronic glaucoma involves no discomfort and only slight visual loss in the early stages and may be well advanced before it is recognized.

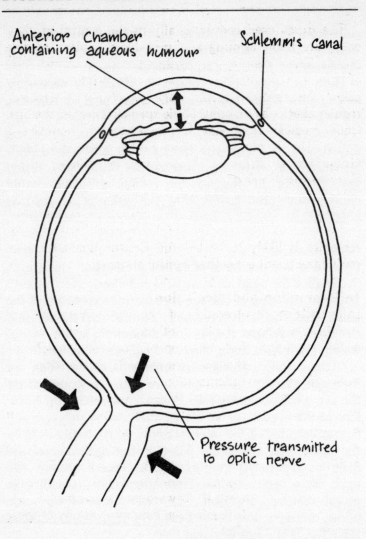

Anterior Chamber containing aqueous humour

Schlemm's canal

Pressure transmitted to optic nerve

A common feature of many types of glaucoma is constriction of the canal of Schlemm, common in long sight and in high degrees of short sight. This would appear to support Dr Bates' contention that the distortion of the eye's shape in these conditions is not natural, but caused by strain, and points to the importance of relaxed normal eye function.

The drugs used conventionally in the control of glaucoma are habit forming and may have unpleasant side effects. Their use may be inevitable at an advanced stage of chronic glaucoma, but can be avoided if it is tackled by gentler means at an earlier stage. If only for this reason, regular checks by an ophthalmic specialist are worthwhile. Once medical treatment has commenced, however, a patient should always continue under a doctor's supervision. Simply throwing away drugs (or glasses) is not recommended; one must work patiently and intelligently for gradual withdrawal as the situation improves.

Emotional factors appear to be important in glaucoma, so working on the emotional picture with Bach flower remedies is likely to be helpful. Constitutional homoeopathic treatment is another fruitful approach.

Inflammation and ulceration

Inflammation or ulceration of the eye is very serious. Anything ending in -itis is an inflammation, hence:

- *Conjunctivitis* Inflammation of the lining membrane that seals the eyeball into the socket.
- *Scleritis* Inflammation of the outer tunic (the white) of the eye.
- *Keratitis* Inflammation of the cornea.
- *Uveitis* The uvea is the layer of the eyeball
- *Choroiditis* between the sclera and the retina, its
- *Iritis* rear part being the choroid, which supports and nourishes the retina, while its forward part is the iris.
  Inflammation can occur at any of these sites.
- *Retinitis* Inflammation of the retina (not to be confused with retinitis pigmentosa – see below).
- *Optic neuritis* Inflammation of the optic nerve. (See diagram page 86.)

Ulcers arise either out of inflammation or from suppurative degenerative conditions. Medical treatment – principally the use of steroid drugs – aims at controlling the

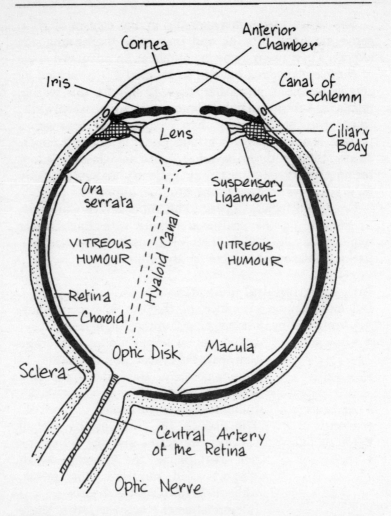

symptoms rather than curing the causes; all the same, it may be valuable in an emergency.

Bathing the eyes is not particularly useful; the best means of cleansing is by natural watering, which can be encouraged by resting and using the eyes in a relaxed way. However, if the eyes are particularly sticky or dry, a weak lukewarm solution of salt in cool boiled water will be better than proprietary solutions. For the long term, careful constitutional homoeopathic treatment will reduce the susceptibility. Detoxification of the body through diet and cleansing regimes, and re-education to normalise the use of the eyes, are also important.

Disease and damage to the retina

In order to fulfil its purpose the *retina* is very delicately constructed, and its powers of regeneration after serious damage are possibly the least of any body tissue. The entire eye and its surroundings are arranged so as to protect the health of the retina as far as possible, so a breakdown is evidence that things have gone very wrong.

Retinitis pigmentosa (RP), contrary to its name, is a non-inflammatory condition involving progressive degeneration of the retinal cells so that they cease to act as photoreceptors. During this process they change colour – hence the name. The loss of vision is gradual, from the periphery inwards, and is irreversible; although it is unlikely to progress to complete blindness, it can go to an extreme of tunnel vision. Night vision will be severely impaired before daylight vision is affected, as more rod cells are involved initially. There is no effective medical treatment; instead clinical care concentrates on low-vision management.

Although the predisposition to retinitis pigmentosa appears to be inherited, the time of onset and rate of visual loss vary enormously. Support for the health generally is clearly important, and this is an area where vitamin therapy may be useful; there is no compelling evidence of benefit from any particular regime, but muscle testing for vitamin need would be an obvious way to explore the question. In visual re-education, emphasising the awareness, without strain, of the periphery of vision and its connection to the other senses may be helpful in both coping with and limiting any visual loss.

Macular degeneration presents the opposite case to RP, in that the macula, the seat of central vision, is damaged first, subsequent visual loss spreading outwards from the centre. It is painless and, in the early stages, will be apparent only from clinical examination or possibly from slight difficulty in dim light. Medical management is mainly confined to monitoring progress and prescribing low-vision aids.

Apart from occurring in the elderly as part of a general picture of senile degeneration, macular disease, like retinal trauma (see below), is most common among people who are very shortsighted. Since, according to Dr Bates, a high level of myopia will involve great strain on the eye and loss of central fixation, it is reasonable to suggest that these factors increase vulnerability to the condition, which also clearly involves a susceptibility to degenerative disease in general. Although possibly incurable in itself, macular degeneration should therefore be regarded as an ultimate development in a process that is entirely preventable and curable in its earlier stages.

Once established, it can help considerably if it is possible to develop a positive joyous hopeful attitude; being able to enjoy the benefit of sight, however limited, leads in time to overcoming the strain and fatigue that arise from the central obstruction. In some places it is considered best to work with the fact that one can see better 'off centre', and try to develop an 'alternative macula'. I have personally preferred to work with whatever is left of the macular vision, because it is clear to me from Dr Bates' work that the macula needs to be fed with relaxed attention, and that its breakdown is due, as much as anything, to strain and neglect. In one case, after a few hours of frustration, I managed to persuade one young man to attend easily and directly to his central blur instead of straining to avoid it. He suddenly became very excited and reported that at the very centre there was a small circle of clear vision – the fovea was intact. By using this in a relaxed and mobile way and allowing it to integrate with the side vision, the overall sight was greatly improved. So, even with the hopeless and 'incurable', it is worth sticking to principle and seeing what can be done.

Retinal trauma takes three basic forms.
- Haemorrhage – rupture of a blood vessel.
- Thrombosis – obstruction of a blood vessel.
- Detachment or tearing of the retina itself.

All these problems are more common amongst those with a high degree of shortsightedness, owing to the strain involved in the elongation of the eye – further evidence for Dr Bates' view that this is not simply a structural abnormality.

In retinal trauma, haemorrhage or detachment can occur spontaneously, but the risk is greatly increased by violent activity or any blow to the head. Ruptures of small blood vessels (capillaries) will not cause much inconvenience once the blood has been absorbed, but larger haemorrhages, or small thromboses (blockages), can damage nervous tissue, resulting in scotomas or blind spots. Damage to or blocking of the main retinal blood vessels results in blindness of that eye.

Detachment of the retina is seldom complete; it usually tears, allowing a small portion to hang loose. Seeing stars following a blow to the head is a result of direct stimulation to the retina and optic nerve; tearing of the retina produces a similar sensation, but more intense and prolonged. Subsequently, the vision becomes disturbingly chaotic, as the folded torn retina transmits random sensations.

Retinal surgery has been transformed by the introduction of laser techniques, but any success in any of these accidents depends on speed and good luck. In any case of a severe blow to the head or obvious injury to the eye, *Arnica* in homoeopathic potency should be taken as soon as possible (if there is great terror and agitation, *Aconite* would be an alternative), and the advice of a homoeopath should be sought and treatment continued – including during and after any surgery – as long as necessary. With retinal detachment, complete rest of the eyes by palming is advisable, and some suggest lying face down.

Proper relaxed use of the eyes minimises the risk of such damage. People with advanced or progressive myopia, especially, need to learn that, in this case at least, prevention is very much the better part of cure.

ASTHENOPIA – VISUAL DISCOMFORT

Visual discomfort, takes many forms, ranging from the simple sensation of eye strain to mind-numbing migraines. The conventional assumption is that strain arises from attempting to use incurably faulty eyes without the benefit of correction, and that it will be cured by glasses. But this is refuted by Dr Bates, who insisted that both discomfort and/or faulty vision result from strain or misuse and that both would be cured by learning to use the eyes normally.

Some people suffer intense pain from using the eyes, while seeing quite normally. One woman who had suffered from years of migraine quite suddenly became myopic, at which point the pain stopped. She described her poor vision as 'like a painless migraine'; clearly the same strain pattern had found a different pathway.

At least as much discomfort is created by wearing glasses as by not wearing them. One short-sighted teenager had suffered from migraines at least once a week for as long as he could remember. After starting Bates lessons and leaving his glasses off, the migraines became very rare, although his vision was still well below normal. Over an active summer vacation he put his glasses away, with no problems of any kind. Wearing them, for his first day back at school prompted an attack, which made him physically sick. In many less dramatic cases there may be a slight error of convergence (easily corrected) to account for the constant headaches, or the sense of strain may be quite undefinable. In most cases relaxing and normalising the visual behaviour does the trick.

In working with vision over a few years I have come to realise something of the marvellous complexity of the human head. The eye muscles exist, not in isolation, but as integral components of the total structure of the face, head and neck, and the excessive tension characterising poor sight is often not confined to the eyes, but involves the related muscles as well. The relief of neck and shoulder tensions by massage, correction of spinal problems or delicate cranial adjustment and improvement of the overall use through the Alexander Technique can all have startling effects on vision. Conversely, working with Dr Bates' techniques to release tensions in the eyes frequently triggers curious reactions in the associated muscles of the face and cranium. Such releases can themselves lead to a degree of discomfort, and it is important to distinguish clearly between such 'growing pains' which may arise from getting it right, and symptoms of increased strain due to getting it wrong.

'Strain pains' are likely to ache, stab or throb; they will probably be relieved by rest – palming – possibly after an initial aggravation of the pain. 'Release pains' commonly involve itching and stinging, spasmodic twitching and, frequently, watering of the eyes; they are irritating rather than genuinely painful, and may be likened to the pins and needles that announce circulation and life returning to a cramped arm or leg. It is best to let these latter pains run their course without interference.

Watering of the eyes is commonly thought of as a problem. But remember that the tears cleanse and protect the surface of the eye and, while wet eyes may be a little inconvenient, it is excessively dry eyes that will be prone to infection. Strain and tension cause the eyes to dry up so, in working for release, an occasional 'cloudburst' is a common and welcome results.

Obviously, pain in the head or eyes may have a variety of other causes, some of them sinister. Before undergoing batteries of tests and complicated treatments, however, it is worthwhile to try just resting the eyes and learning to use them normally. If the problem is relieved in this way it is reasonable to assume that strain alone was the culprit and that, together with the symptoms, the cause has been removed.

7
THE FIRST CONSULTATION

You may receive vision education from a specialist Bates teacher working alone and at home, or perhaps in a natural health centre; or you may be taught by an optometrist or even a medical practitioner. In at least two states of the USA medical supervision is a legal requirement, in others independent Bates teachers can work freely, on the basis that their work is *educational* and they do not trespass on the territory of optometrist or doctor. In Europe there is a mixed community of optometrically and educationally qualified practitioners. Some teachers may combine vision education work with other forms of education or healing. None of this makes any difference provided you have confidence in your teacher, and at least you can be sure that no-one has taken up the Bates work as a path to easy popularity or a quick fortune!

Take your current glasses to the first visit along with copies, if you have them, of any prescriptions, medical reports etc. If you use contact lenses, be prepared to take them out!

The first consultation has four main objectives:
- Taking a *history* of the case.
- Making an *assessment* of the vision.
- Agreeing a *contract*.
- Beginning *work* as appropriate.

Different teachers will vary in their priorities and in their methods – no two consultations are alike. I allow one and a half hours for the whole procedure and find that usually works well.

TAKING A HISTORY

The optician is interested mainly in your eyes. In contrast the Bates teacher is concerned with *you* and how you see. The initial discussion may therefore cover quite a lot of ground.

Concerning your vision, we will want to know:
- Status – nature of the problem.
- Onset – when problems began.
- Progress – how they have developed.

More generally we like to know about:
- Eyes – injuries or disease.
- Head injuries, concussion, etc.
- Headaches and migraine.
- Spinal injuries or problems.
- Health in general – any chronic or recurring problems.
- Medications used – present or past.
- Surgery under anaesthetic.
- Substance use/abuse (alcohol, tobacco, etc.).

There are practical reasons for all of this. Apart from direct or indirect relevance to the state of the sight, it is important to know of circumstances that might make particular practices inadvisable, e.g. spinal injuries or balance problems.

More generally still, you may be asked about:
- Work.
- Family/social life.
- Recreations, sport and hobbies.

This is not idle curiosity or just making conversation. Insight into your personality helps to understand the visual problem and the best approach to it. Knowledge of your lifestyle makes it easier to suggest appropriate ways of incorporating what you will learn into your daily life. But there is never any intention to invade privacy, and if you do not wish to discuss any particular aspect of your life – no problem.

MAKING AN ASSESSMENT

A visual profile is formed from the individual assessments of different areas and a study of their relationships. The techniques used are more than somewhat rustic by comparison with the glittering hi-tech of the eye clinic, but they do their job. Equally importantly, by using simple procedures the pupil is much better able to follow what is happening and to feel involved. Since we are not attempting to prescribe lenses or to carry out surgery, and since the condition of the sight is likely to vary, pinpoint measurement is neither necessary nor useful – we simply want to find out what is going on.

Acuity testing is carried out in the usual way using test cards for distant and near vision (see pages 148–51). Since this first acuity 'score' forms the baseline against which future improvement will be judged, I always err on the side of recording the best level possible, if there is any doubt.

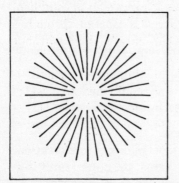 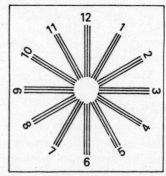

Clock dials used in assessing astigmatism

When taking the test, the most important thing is *not to try*. Just relax, breathe normally and let your eyes move easily around the chart, naming (or guessing at?) any letters that look familiar. It's no crime to read them in the wrong order, and guessing at a half-recognised letter is not 'cheating' but intelligence. By all means discuss *how* the letters appear, as well as naming them. Remember also that you are not necessarily supposed to be able to read the bottom line – don't worry about what you should be seeing, just report what you do see. The Bates method is all about looking without strain, so start as you mean to go on.

- *Astigmatism* is assessed using clock dials. Precise measurement is less important than comparison between the eyes and the degree of stability/mobility.
- *Photophobia* (intolerance of light) and the pupillary reflex (action of the iris) are simply checked using a flashlight.
- *Peripheral* field (side vision) can be estimated by noting the limits of awareness of a white card. 'Colour fields' may be noted in some cases.
- *Tracking* (accuracy of pursuits and vergences, see pages 53–8) can be estimated by watching the eyes track a moving target – a pencil point or flashlight. Together with the objective accuracy of movement, any sensations of strain or discomfort are noted.
- *Dominance* (preference for the leading eye) is established with a screen test. (A target is located through a small hole in a screen – this can only be done with one eye.)
- *Fusion* (present or absence of binocular vision) is checked using a 'nosecard' and confirmed in case of doubt by other binocularity techniques (see page 112).

Merging these separate assessments into a profile of visual function will throw up a number of interesting questions, for example:

- Is the dominant eye more or less acute?
- Is astigmatism stable or variable?
- Does the acuity change during testing?
- Is a squint one-sided or alternating?
- How does the objective information compare with subjective experience? And with the history?

A TYPICAL CASE SHEET

In studying a case, the vision educator's job is to make sense of the relationship between the various factors, in contrast with the orthodox approach which often either considers each bit of the problem separately or simply assumes that a fixed relationship exists.

In relation to the acuity and refraction, the rate of progression is obviously of as much interest as the present condition; someone who had normal vision up to the age of 20 and is then in six dioptre glasses by 22 is obviously a slightly different case from someone with similar vision who has been wearing glasses since the age of six. If there is a big difference in acuity between the eyes is is often significant whether the better or worse eye is dominant. (It is quite possible for an eye which is so nearsighted as to be almost blind to be dominant even though its partner eye sees normally.) A dominant 'good' eye tends to indicate that the imbalance is caused by strain, while a dominant 'poor' eye would suggest genuine 'laziness', or disconnection. Although similar techniques will be used in either case, there is obviously a difference of emphasis in the way they will be applied. The relationship between near and far vision needs to be considered. If the near vision is unusually good or bad for a given level of distance vision, one would suspect that the ability to change focus might be impaired, and that this might be more important than the basic resting focus. Reading difficulties can be especially interesting; as well as the focus of the eyes, we have to consider the convergence (it helps if both eyes look at the same thing) and also all the movements of the eyes. Many people have suffered from being forced to read too early and, although they can do it, always associate it with a sense of strain and effort which then extends to the entire way they use their eyes. This will often show up in erratic tracking movements or a sense of discomfort when the eyes are required to move.

It is very common to find all sorts of problems in relation to binocular seeing of which the pupil was completely unaware. Many people have errors of conver-

---

A. Myope ♂ 23   dob 4.10.67.

1 Thatstreet
Thistown, tel 121212
Whatshire

History
Short sight: onset age 11. Specs since age 12 — wears
  permanently.
Since 3 yrs incr. headache, eyestr. + vision deteriorated.
Eyes ok. Head ok.
Spine? Strained back at work.
Gen health ok — no medication.
Occ. clerk/storekeeper
M. 1 child age 3. Some dom. tension — broken nights etc.

Assess   astig   R ☀ L ☀ B ☀

    6m   14″   phot mild   pr slow

R   6/24   36%   track ✓ strain conv⁺ ←—»

L   6/36   27%   sv 165° ∨

B   6/18   48%   dom L   hand R

                fus ? responds to colours

[A Typical Case Sheet]

gence, not big enough to be called a squint but big
enough to make a significant contribution to the blur they
see and to cause discomfort. Then there are the imbalances in the 'signal strength' from the eyes to the brain,
although these may be thought of mainly as a perceptual
problem they also have consequences for the balanced (or
not) use of the muscles. Then there is the vexing question
of the relationship between the visual difficulty and other
issues of physical, mental and emotional health. It may be
appropriate to think of referring the pupil for some other
form of help, either alongside the Bates work or even given

priority over it. This may or may not accord with the wishes of the pupil who may be very open to working on the vision in a broad based way, or may take the rather narrow view that they have come to do 'eye exercises' and no more or less.

THE 'CONTRACT'

All this is before we get to the point of dealing with the pupil's expectations regarding time, cost, and the degree of improvement to be expected, which may be entirely realistic and positive, and then again may not. There are actually some people who, having abused their eyes for sixty years will be seriously upset if they do not experience a massive improvement on their first visit. Others appear to have no real expectation of anything happening at all and are quite alarmed if it does! Accordingly some people find the cost and commitment involved utterly outrageous, or want guarantees of definite progress within a very short time span, others would see it as remarkably good value and are quite happy to attend lessons for years for the fun of it. I (and, I would hope, my colleages) invariably try to share my understanding of the situation, such as it is, as fully as possible, and to be as realistic as possible about what is needed and what I think will happen. It is obviously important to get this straight from the beginning to avoid misunderstanding and later unhappiness.

The questions which most commonly occur at this point are:

Will vision actually become normal, or just 'better'?

Does it become 'automatic' or will I always have to work at it?

What rate of progress can be expected?

When vision has been deteriorating for years, to change the situation in any sense for the better is a considerable achievement. Realistically the goals are:

a) stabilise – arrest deterioration

b) improve – as far as possible
c) normalise – if possible

Only normal vision, by definition, is effortlessly self-regulating and completely stable, Normality is therefore the ultimate goal, although there can be a big difference between 'almost' and absolutely. The most one can say is that if the eyes and mind are encouraged to function normally, vision will be as good as physiologically possible. The closer one can get to normality the less conscious attention will be needed to maintain the direction of improvement so it is always worth working for rapid progress in the early stages.

STARTING WORK

As a generalisation, I expect to take 6–10 sessions to cover the basic ground, and to make significant discoveries and/ or progress in that time. Beyond that it is hard to say, some people progress amazingly rapidly others less so. My speed record was two weeks to complete relief of a squint case but that was rather the exception!

I prefer to see pupils at least weekly at first to maintain continuity and momentum. Meeting less frequently puts a great onus on the pupil, which only a few can live up to, to maintain motivation. Children can respond very well, however, and often need less attention than adults. At the other extreme, intensive courses can be very productive. I occasionally take residential pupils for a week or so and, although requiring stamina on both sides, this can be very worthwhile. Some of the basic techniques can be taught in a group setting and working in a group can be stimulating and fun. However, the most important difficulties encountered will always be individual and not to be overcome except with the close personal attention received in a course of private lessons.

The practical part of the first session is not supposed to perform any miracles, but to enable the pupil to start thinking about the seeing process while getting into a condition in which the real work can have some effect. We

begin therefore with the elements of hygiene, an introduction to the practice of resting the eyes as an approach
to relaxation, and one or two simple exercises to begin to
develop the perception. It is then possible to go on to
introduce further concepts and techniques in the most
appropriate order for the individual situation. I usually
like to make at least some progress towards bringing the
eyes into balance and alignment a first priority because it
makes everything else so much easier, but it really
depends very much on the individual case.

A really clear understanding of what we are doing only
comes about through experience over time, but I am
always at pains to make clear from the very beginning that
we are *not*:

- doing physical exercises
- trying to strengthen muscles
- making the eyes work harder

but that we *are*:

- developing relaxed perception
- learning to use the eyes without strain

There are still some people who suffer fixed ideas on this
point and do not seem to grasp the real idea however often
it is discussed, but we do our best.

One has to remember that the rate of progress does not
depend on doing set exercises for x minutes per day, but
on the ability to change. When asked how much time one
should give, I point out that for all the time the eyes are
open one is either choosing to use them well, or allowing
them to be misused by default. It is only possible to
improve when the lessons learned are incorporated into
the daily round. The patterns and rates of improvement
are as individual as the means used to bring it about.
There may be a slow, steady improvement – the blur
gradually clears, the squint eye slowly lessens its deviation; or there may be flashes – the eye straightens, the
vision clears for a second or two, and then reverts. A
common experience involves both kinds of improvement

converging; as the 'baseline' situation improves, so the 'flashes' of normality become longer and more frequent. The overall timescale can range from minutes to years.

Mechanical repetition of 'exercises' will change nothing. Every exercise, properly understood, is an experiment or demonstration, which makes clear the nature of available choices. The important part is learning to recognise the choices and to choose what is most helpful. Many people understand this quite easily. Others, having been brought up in the belief that only strenuous effort brings rewards and that struggle is virtuous, will come to it more slowly. When they do, they will find they have acquired much more than better vision.

A particularly vexing question is the measurement of improvement. One might think that the answer would be to visit the optician periodically for an eye test but, certainly in the short term, this is not always reliable. The testing process is notorious for lowering the vision and, particularly for people in the early stages of vision education, can produce completely perverse results. This is because the first aim is always to move from a state which is fixed, with the eyes not responding to anything particularly, to one where the eyes are sensitive and responsive. This sensitivity is rather double-edged, vision will suffer under adverse circumstances as well as improve under beneficial conditions. Developing a reliably stable and robust co-ordination which will operate under any kind of duress is another matter, particularly for those who have suffered poor sight for many years. To take a simple analogy: two children practising the piano may play a particular piece equally well nine times out of ten. Asked to play in a school concert, one will still play well, the other will go to pieces with nerves. It would be grossly unfair and unintelligent to say that the nervous child cannot really play the piece, since there are occasions when he does so, and may even play it a great deal more beautifully than the reliable performer. It could be even more stupid to assert that the nervous one had something wrong with his fingers which prevented him from playing.

101

But it is clear that some further steps are needed to become a competent performer.

In exactly the same way, I have known people who have experienced great improvement in their everyday vision and yet were devastated to have an optician tell them that their sight had got worse. In fact it had become more variable, and was at its best much better, but the test had brought out the worst. By definition, one would expect people who have experience of vision problems to be 'nervous performers' in this sense so this has to be allowed for.

This was well illustrated by a recent case. A young boy whom I had seen two years earlier was brought to see me. At our previous meeting he had been so very slightly myopic that I had advised no particular action. He had had no difficulties seeing and had been quite happy meanwhile. He then saw an optician who found his vision four times worse than previously and insisted that he

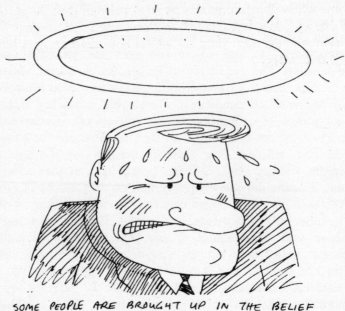

SOME PEOPLE ARE BROUGHT UP IN THE BELIEF THAT STRUGGLE IS VIRTUOUS

immediately have strong glasses and wear them all the time, scolding the mother for neglecting her child. One month later at a routine test at school he found he could not read the chart with his glasses but could do so perfectly well without. His (rather confused) mother asked me to see him again and I found his vision perfectly normal. When asked, he recalled that on the day of the sight test it had been extremely hot and he had had a difficult day at school, he had been hot and thirsty while they had waited for half an hour to be seen, and the optician, who was behind in his appointments, had been rather brusque! To me, this explained the situation quite well: his normal vision had reacted quite normally to stressful circumstances and produced a test result which, although valid at the time, bore no relation at all to his usual behaviour.

So in general I think it is a good idea not to attach too much importance to test results, and to place more value on the quality of everyday seeing. There will always be some who will interpret this as an admission that the state of the eye does not change and that the improvement in vision is imaginary: they are welcome to their opinion but it is not correct.

8
WHAT, HOW AND WHY

This is not a 'how to' book. A book can explain an idea, but practical skills need to be learned in practice. A book will tell you what, and to some extent why, but only a teacher can show you how.

Many of the techniques originated by Dr Bates and developed by his followers have been described in print more than once. In re-describing a few of them I would wish to show how they fit together in relation to the single principle – that the proper use of the eyes, leading to normal relaxed function, is achieved through balancing the elements of *awareness*, *attention* and *acceptance*, as expressed in the following three affirmations:
- I am *aware* of my surroundings.
- I *attend* to one thing at a time, within my awareness.
- I *accept* unconditionally what I see.

There are few, if any, specific exercises for particular conditions – each exercise is a way of examining particular aspects of seeing, and will play its part in the general process. Trying to concentrate on what is most 'relevant' may be a mistake; often it is the very exercise that seems least appealing/profitable that holds the key to the problem. The teacher, who can take a relatively detached view, must choose the order and priorities, and above all must make sure that the work is thoroughly understood.

EYE HYGIENE

Hygiene of the eyes, like that of all body tissues, is based on the requirements of nutrition and elimination. Both depend in turn on the free circulation of blood and lympatic fluid, which can be enhanced in a number of ways.

- Breathe freely and naturally. Those who strain to see often hold an attitude of tense concentration. This robs the eyes of oxygen, making it harder to see. Don't do deep breathing exercises, however; listen to your breathing, and let it find its own relaxed rhythm.
- Blink freely and blink often. Rapid light blinks and 'big fat squeezes' moisten and cleanse the eyes, rest them from the light, and enable them to relax, change and become mobile.
- Splash the eyes with water (keeping the eyes closed) to stimulate blood circulation. Alternate groups of hot and cold (or warm and cool) splashes. But note that, for eye disease patients and those with very poor sight, it will be better to bathe the closed eyelids lightly with a sponge or flannel.
- Bouncing gently (on a small trampoline), or similar gentle exercise, is good for stimulating the lymph drainage, helping to remove toxins.

PALMING – REST AND RELAXATION

The purpose of palming is to allow the eyes to rest, as the basis for the experience of relaxation. In palming, the hands, slightly cupped, cover the eye sockets, with the fingers crossed on the forehead. The eyes are closed, and are carefully covered to exclude all light. There may be firm contact between hands and face, but there should be none at all between the hands and eyes. The elbows should be supported so that the back is comfortably straight and there is no undue pressure on the neck, shoulders and arms.

Palming has a number of purposes, the foremost of which is to rest the eyes. We sit down to rest our feet when we feel the need; similarly if the eyes are accepted as part of the living body, it will be understood that they, too, need rest occasionally. When the sight is perfectly normal the eyes work easily and need very little rest; but when sight is

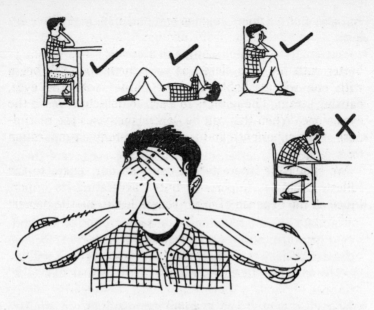

abnormal due to strain, all activity is relatively tiring, so more rest is needed. Any symptoms of strain, soreness, itchiness of the eyes, many headaches and general weariness are usually indications to rest by palming. The more quickly one responds to, or even anticipates, these needs, the less resting time will be required.

Relaxation of mind and body can be well developed through palming. Relaxation does not mean switching off and collapsing, but releasing tension and behaving as required in the most appropriate economical balanced way. The eye is only free from strain when it is used correctly, by central fixation, so relaxation in Dr Bates' sense equates to good use and normal coordination. Palming is a special case since, as there is no sensory input, the proper activity of the eye is to do nothing. This in turn provides a reference point from which strain in everyday activities will be more easily recognised, which is the first step towards its prevention.

Thinking and sensing
Creative mental activity is a valuable extension of palming.

All kinds of exercises in memory and imagination, every kind of mental task, from arranging a shopping list to composing a symphony, can be carried out just as easily or better with the eyes closed as with them open. To begin with one will probably tend to 'think' with the eyes, causing strain. The point is to learn to detach, to leave the eyes alone. When this can be done it increases the restfulness of the experience and makes it a valuable preparation for seeing.

We should be interested in using all our senses to the fullest. Seeing is important, but exaggerating its importance at the expense of other senses leaves us the poorer; and it is also counterproductive, because the sight takes on too much and begins to strain. Accepting that vision is in many respects a secondary sense makes it much easier to use the eyes in a normal and relaxed way, so as to get the best out of them. Palming provides an excellent opportunity to become better acquainted with touch, smell and hearing, even taste, and many useful practices can be developed with the eyes closed.

Exploring these other senses, which are essentially passive, makes it easier to apply discriminating attention without making the effort to do anything, just accepting. In making the transition between eyes closed and eyes open, the important questions concern the relationship between seeing and its companions – for example, does seeing enhance or diminish the experience of the other senses? – and the ability to find, within the seeing sense itself, this balance of doing and non-doing.

GLASSES – ON OR OFF?

If vision is to become normal, or is to change in any way, we have to learn to see without glasses. This does not mean they should always be discarded out of hand – just that their use should be less automatic.

If we consider that the basic purpose of all our senses is to establish contact with our surroundings we are entitled to ask whether wearing glasses helps or hinders that contact. The answer we are likely to find is that it is often a question of attitude. We can be cut off from the experience of our surroundings not only by the blur of poor sight, but also by the mental apathy created by having clear vision 'spoon-fed'.

On the other hand, if we are prepared to enter into our surroundings in a feeling sort of way, then the sense of vital contact may be just as strong regardless of whether the images are clear or blurred.

Of course there are times when clarity is vitally important – if you need your glasses then use them by all means – but let them be an aid to your seeing rather than a substitute for it.

Our object is to avoid strain in seeing, and anyone with chronically poor sight has to realise that he is always straining, more or less, with or without glasses, since otherwise he would see normally. The solution to this dilemma is to recognise that some times the strain will be greater with glasses, at other times without, and to act accordingly. The important thing is to *avoid* the three D's:

- *Difficulty*
- *Discomfort* and, above all
- *Danger*

It is also simply necessary to recognise the times when seeing can be more satisfactory and enjoyable, although less accurate, without glasses. With time the balance will shift inexorably towards less use.

Spectacles versus contact lenses

Contact lenses, where there are no tolerance problems, probably interfere with eye function less than spectacles. Many users have reported that vision seems to deteriorate less rapidly with contact lenses than with spectacles, and there are good optical, physiological and psychological reasons why this may be so.

The drawback is that it is easier to keep contact lenses in than to take them out, and the effortless illusion they create of 'natural vision' can undermine the desire to work for real improvement. For these reasons I support their continued use by pupils whose vision is so poor that they are only occasionally able to manage without. But for anyone who should be able to adopt a more flexible approach, I advise them to use glasses for everyday wear, simply because disliking them is a good incentive to taking them off; they can then reserve the contacts for occasions when appearance and confidence are especially important.

By developing an active interested attitude to seeing at all times, the restrictions on the eyes and the distortions imposed by glasses will probably become more noticeable. As this leads naturally to taking them off more often, the transition between the two levels of vision will become ever easier, especially if palming is used frequently. 'Perfect relaxation' is an ideal; when one is able to see in an *increasingly* relaxed way at all times, with or without glasses, the vision cannot help but improve.

COLOUR INTO FORM

Even for the colour blind, perception of form depends on recognising the different qualities of light reflected from different surfaces; an 'outline' is essentially a change of colour.

Straining at a patch of colour is less likely than straining to read a letter; at least, the uselessness of the effort will quickly become apparent. So we begin with colour as a way of learning to direct the attention spontaneously within the field of awareness, with a relaxed acceptance of what is seen. Noticing a colour as it enters the field of vision cuts through day-dreaming and provides a way of learning that the attention is focused, not by effort, but through a 'crystallisation' of awareness.

However poor the vision at a given distance, different colours can always be discriminated if the areas and contrast are great enough. This immediately transforms the question from the absolute (whether one can see) to the relative (what one can see). Once the 'difficulty' is recognised as relative it is always easy to make further progress.

SPACE AND MOVEMENT – THE SWINGS

The exercises called swings by Dr Bates embody the principle of visual movement. This is crucial to the operation of central fixation as well as the appreciation of spatial relationships, both of these, in turn, being important to accurate focusing. Many different types of swing have been invented, but all are derived from a few basic types.

The purpose of the basic swings is analytical; they are not so much models of proper seeing as artificial ways to explore various aspects individually. They do however have a common theme in continuity of awareness and clear direction of attention.

The sway

In the sway the body swings from side to side while the attention is directed towards a distant point. One becomes aware of the constantly shifting relationships in the field of vision, using the fixation point as a 'pivot'. It is customary to use a nearby reference point such as an upright pole or the glazing bar of a window, to establish the 'movement' initially (see diagram below).

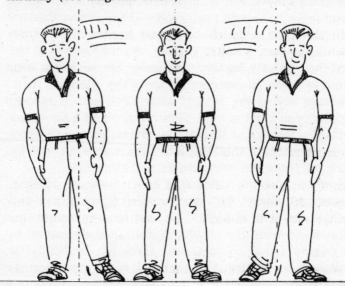

THE SWAY

At first the sway appears to be no more than a demonstration of simple parallax (the apparent change in the spatial relationship of objects viewed from different positions), but, as more relaxed awareness develops, the experience of movement becomes extraordinarily complex which has the effect of relaxing and mobilising the eyes. It then becomes possible to extend the experience by walking backwards and forwards, noticing the apparent coming and going of the surroundings. This can create an awareness of shifts in perspective and a greater sense of centring or grounding in relation to the surroundings. By making distance more meaningful, this helps create the possibility of accurate focusing.

True swings

In the sway the fixation point is static while the body movement creates shifts in the point of view. The true swings have the contrary intention of observing a continuously shifting fixation point from a viewpoint that is, ideally, stationary. The effect of this is that the object/scene appears to pass smoothly in the opposite direction and at the same speed as the actual movement.

- In the *long swing* the eyes, head and body move together.
- In the *head swing* the eyes and head move together, while the body is stationary.
- In the *optical swing* the eyes alone move, while the head and body are stationary.

The idea is always to control the eyes indirectly through the control of the attention. They should not fix on objects, neither must they 'glaze out', looking at nothing. The best approach to the correct attitude is through the sense of touch, allowing the eyes to follow a path as though tracing it with a fingertip. In the early stages it is usually easier to develop this sense of effortless contact by working rather slowly; once it is established, speed is unimportant; one will simply practise in the way that is most relaxing.

- In the *long swing* I prefer a body turn of exactly 180°. Working in a room this makes it easier to check the head/body/eyes alignment as one can square up to a

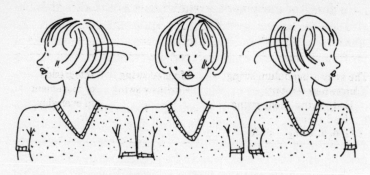

THE HEAD SWING

wall (or mirror) at either end of each swing.

- The *head swing* is limited by how far the neck will turn easily (it is not necessary to use force). Check at each end of the swing that the eyes are pointing the same way as the nose.

- The *optical swing* begins by mimicking the head swing, but with only the eyes allowed to move. The conscious thought is always directed to a movement of the attention that stimulates the eye movement indirectly. As the eyes become more relaxed and mobile, it becomes possible simply to observe a slight vibration of the object regarded, due to the spontaneous movement of the eye. It is then unnecessary to do anything; the appearance or lack of movement can simply to monitored to indicate the decrease or increase of strain.

The drifting swing

Having carefully dissected visual movement into its component parts, the drifting swing puts them all back together again. Head, eyes and body are allowed to move freely in a kind of slow 'disco dance', only the feet remaining still. Rather than directing the eyes to this or that point, the object is scrupulously to leave them alone and observe the results. Those who master this are getting very close to experiencing complete sensory relaxation together with clearly, but effortlessly, focused attention.

Experience of movement – relationship of the swings

Analysis	Synthesis	Integration

The sway – pendulum swing
True swings – rotary
   Body swing – long swing
   Head swing
   Optical swing – shift
	Monkey swing
	– drifting swing
		Integration
		of movement
		in everyday
		life

What do the swings do?

Used intelligently and in combination, the swings, as described, considerably enhance the everyday experience of seeing, through the awareness of change and movement. Establishing a truer sense of one's immediate relationship to the three-dimensional concrete world as an involved participant helps create the mental condition for clearer seeing by freeing the eyes.

BINOCULARITY AND CONVERGENCE TECHNIQUES

Where binocular vision is lacking, putting it back together is generally a high priority, and, in my own experience, is nearly always possible, given time and provided that there is no damage to eye, nerve or brain. The case analysis will work out the relationship between the suppression and factors such as squint and anisometropia (when the focusing of each eye is different, see page 70). In some cases it may be necessary to take the circular route, juggling all the factors, but if it is possible to establish binocular vision as a first step, it usually makes life easier. Once that is achieved it is then possible to work on normalising the convergence; if convergence inaccuracy can be eliminated as a source of blur, it is then possible to work on the acuity. All very neat in theory – and occasionally so in practice.

The basic requirement is for instruments that will give

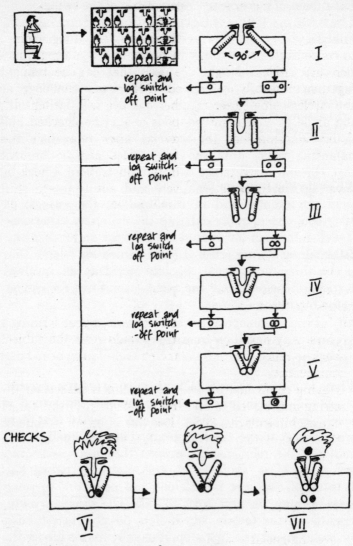

Binocularity work-up flow chart.

feedback on what is happening. Ours are very simple, comprising two 6-inch cardboard tubes, a 20-foot length of string and some coloured clips, and two knitting needles. Yes, really!

Binocularity work-up – cardboard tubes

The tubes are used as binoculars, completely covering the eyes. Regard a blank surface or the sky, and don't attempt to concentrate on anything in particular. In normal function two circles of light are seen that can be brought together until fully overlapped. If there is a challenge, as the circles come closer together one eye will 'switch off'; the angle at which this happens should be checked and noted. Recommence the exercise after relaxation and balancing work, until the two circles can be brought together and fused (stage V in the illustration). Check by covering the tubes alternatively and noting image shift (VI) and merging colours of two different coloured balls (VII), then proceed to the string.

Binocularity and convergence work-up – the string

A length of string, fixed to a point 20 feet away, or less, is held up to the nose.

- If function is binocular, two strings will appear forming a cross. Any deviation from this should refer the subject back to relaxation and balancing techniques, or to basic binocularity.
- Having confirmed binocularity, a clip is placed on the string and moved to and fro. If attention to this target causes binocularity to fail, it is due to strain. Reinforce the binocularity and use relaxation (palming, with appropriate visualisations). If binocularity holds but convergence is inaccurate, this can usually be corrected by visualisation.
- Three or more clips on the string will form patterns as indicated, with the clip regarded at the centre of the cross and clearly single.

The string thus gives feedback in three areas:

- Binocularity and balance (check that the two strings are equally 'solid').
- Accuracy of convergence (check that the target is single and is at the centre of the cross).
- Integration of central/peripheral vision (check that the

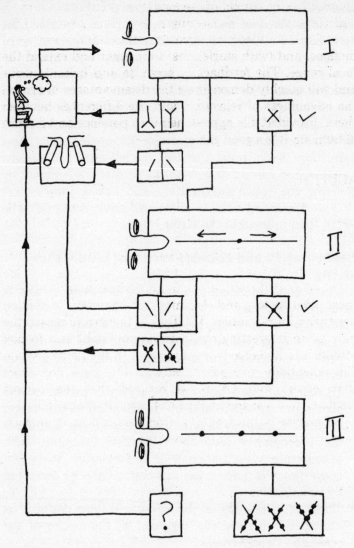

Convergence and balance work-up flow chart.

subject is easily able to see pairs of clips peripherally in
the foreground and background).

The advantage of the string is that it is continuous; it
condenses, so to speak, a filament of space, enabling us to

monitor the movement of the eyes from point to point in its entirety instead of registering a leap. It is also used for assessing the speed of accommodation and convergent motions, and (with single eyes) to monitor and extend the focal range. The feedback is accurate and instantaneous and will quickly demonstrate the disadvantages of strain, the advantages of relaxation and the differences between them. Provided it is approached with patience and a sense of humour, it is a good game.

ACUITY

In order for blurs to become clear we have to make the best use of the feedback between eye and brain. In chronic poor sight the presence of the blur actually stimulates unhelpful reactions that reduce the feedback either by strain to see better or by giving up/switching off.

Improving acuity requires finding the 'equator' between these two poles and learning to maintain attention together with relaxation. The trick is to learn to regard the blur as an interesting object in its own right and to pay attention to its behaviour. Any object in the field of vision can potentially give good feedback, but some give more than others and Dr Bates realised that the perfect feedback tool was the Snellen test card (see page 150).

So precise is the feedback from the test card, in fact, that it becomes a very powerful stimulus to misuse. Everyone who has visited an optician will recall the anxiety and strain to read the 'bottom line', compounded of fear about the state of their sight and the wish to please, to 'pass' the test. The first stage in progress, then, is to recognise this reaction for what it is and to learn to control – to inhibit – it. That is why the concept of acceptance is so important.

I have found it helpful to expand the range of the chart by adding some plain coloured cards, a card with smaller test type on it and a near-vision reading card. The colours require no effort to see them, and the tiny letters on the smaller test card make the futility of effort obvious, even

117

to the most stubborn trier, as well as emphasising the important difference between visible and legible. Far too often pupils will say 'I can't see anything' when of course they mean 'I can't read anything'.

Movement is important. Practising a swing with the chart in view will often produce a quick result to get the feedback ball rolling. When the eyes are working fairly well, the natural shift begins to operate; looking steadily but easily at a small letter we can see it vibrate or pulsate and become clearer as it does so. A moving blur is always more interesting than a static one and I always recommend giving priority of attention to the movement aspect. This creates a situation in which clarity can develop, whereas direct attempts to achieve clarity are counterproductive.

Working with alternate eyes is very important. Dissociating the eyes always increases strain at first, reducing the vision and threatening to induce the vicious circle. Learning to recognize and deal with that leads to great improvement when the eyes are used together.

Acceptance does not mean fatalism about the state of the sight – learning to live with it. On the contrary, it means actively entering into the experience of the present – the only point from which we can achieve change. Once the chart is looked at in this accepting attentive way, without fear or strain, it can begin to do its proper job. Simply by noticing that at some moments it looks clearer than at others, one is acknowledging and encouraging the learning process. If it becomes especially clear as a result of a particular practice – palming or swinging, say – then the link is subconsciously as well as consciously established between the sensations of relaxation and movement and the experience of clearer sight. All kinds of strategies can be devised to practise looking at the chart with continuous interest while avoiding strain: different ways of sequencing the letters; different patterns of breathing or of opening the eyes; combinations with swings, with near and far shifts. The list is endless, and the inventiveness of the individual teacher comes into play in helping the pupil to find the right balance.

Whatever technique is used, certain factors are always important:

- *Distance.*
- *Neutrality.*
- *Illumination.*
- *Memory* and *imagination.*

Distance

It is a good idea to work from a distance such that every character on the chart can be seen as a separate shape. It is a question of giving the mind something to go on. Too close, and the exercise is pointless: too far and we run the risk of giving up and losing mental contact, or of straining hopelessly.

Neutrality

Letters that are 'impossible' to read should be looked at in exactly the same frame of mind as those that are easy to read. The whole basis of using the test card is that the reducing sizes of letters provide stepping stones to greater acuity within a continuum. Preconceptions such as 'That one's obvious' (don't bother) and 'That one's too hard' (don't try) get in the way.

Illumination

At first one should work with the best available light. When good results are consistently obtained, practice in lower light levels will be helpful.

The light level affects the situation in a number of ways. Basically, we are concerned with processing information. More light, more information – simple. Then there is the function of the iris which contracts in bright light (the pupilary reflex). This is not, as is often thought, to protect the eye from light, but to make the best use of available light. This is achieved in two ways. Firstly, reducing the aperture means that the light entering the eye becomes relatively coherent, the effect of errors of refraction is reduced and the blur circle made smaller. Secondly, the depth of field is increased, making the discrimination of an object as in/out of focus more critical. The combined effect of these two factors is to increase dramatically the quality of useful information to the brain; even a small increase in light can improve both quality and quantity of information, to the point where a torpid visual system feels obliged to do something with it. Once the pump is primed in this way and information is flowing, the light can be reduced very substantially while maintaining much the same level of vision.

Memory and imagination

Memory and imagination are tools as vital now as they were for Dr Bates, and it is important to understand their use in the correct positive light. To compare something with how it looked before is not to be confused with passing judgement, trying to do better; it is a way of checking the quality of perception, since a meaningful comparison between two experiences can only be made if both have been absorbed in a relaxed and dispassionate way. Similarly, use of the imagination to project future possibilities is in no way wishful thinking or self-deception; it is a matter of identifying different options so as to be able to choose between them.

In addition to formal exercises, it is therefore useful to have a test card around, placed strategically where one will pass it regularly at a convenient distance. At first the temptation is to 'test' all the time (Am I better yet?). Cancel that thought, or wait until the novelty wears off, then just use the chart as a casual reminder of being involved in the process of working with vision – constant evidence that the sight is always changing and as an occasional source of pleasant surprises.

It occasionally happens that people who experience good results when working with the test card find their sight resistant to change at other times. It is all a question of applying the lessons learned, of taking the same kind of active interest and looking for the same kind of progression from large to small details with the same kind of openness to change. The test card is clear and unambiguous, but it is also not intrinsically very interesting. The world is much more interesting and filled with ambiguity. Making the transition from one to the other a matter of patience and practice.

It also happens that someone who practises an exercise without apparent success will 'coincidentally' experience a massive improvement in vision shortly afterwards. Improvement requires two things – improving the information flow, and not straining. Most people strain to some extent while practising an exercise, however much they intend to relax. This will limit the result at that time, but it will not prevent information from being taken in and processed. At another time, when one is more spontaneously relaxed – typically at times when, as we say, 'something catches the eye' – it is put to use.

One lady drove me to despair by an apparent total failure to react or benefit in any way from some weeks of work. Then, as a casual aside, she revealed that for everyday purposes her sight had improved fantastically. When I remonstrated, she said 'But you only asked me when we were doing exercises and they always make it worse – but it's fine now!' *Nil desperandum.*

Near-point acuity
Near-point acuity is approached in the same way as for distance. Everybody works on this aspect – it is as important to the person with short sight who needs to extend range outwards as to the person with long sight needing to extend inwards. It also offers the possibility of directly using the sense of touch.

The simple act of tracing with a pointer or needle leads directly to the correct use of the attention – to one point at a time. One does not need to 'concentrate' on the point; the fact that it is there is enough. Physically practising like this at the near point also becomes a basis for the imaginative use of 'touch' at the distance, which is absolutely necessary in understanding the swings. My favourite device for starting near-point work is an Ordnance Survey map. Most people find maps an even bigger headache than test cards, so learning to use them for relaxation is profitable and fun. The combination of coloured graphics and text in all kinds of sizes enables the map to work like a randomised test card, with a more balanced appeal to the two brain hemispheres.

Once contact is established at the reading distance, books, magazines and newspapers can be used. Patience is the greatest virtue – an unhurried relaxed approach always brings dividends. It is good to begin by absolutely refusing to try to read, instead studying the text as though it were an abstract pattern – a piece of carpet or some wallpaper. If words begin to clarify, don't be greedy to absorb their meaning; instead concentrate on the appearance. If the point is reached where the words are clear and meaning is apparent, again, don't be greedy – pause, rest and reflect. This is a good strategy in any kind of reading problem, not just those connected with focusing.

Above all, treat any blurring not as a 'nuisance', to be overcome, but as information about what you are doing that you can learn to use. A successful approach is always one that is less concerned with the immediate end result and more interested in the process.

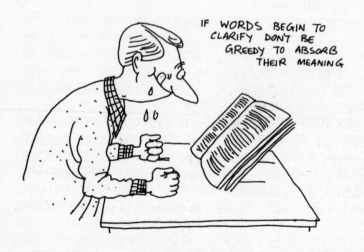

HAND AND EYE

The development of physical coordination is an invaluable part of learning to see. As mentioned earlier, sight develops as a secondary adjunct to more direct ways of learning about the world. To insist on touch as the primary sense is a useful corrective in a culture whose first law is look but don't touch. Looking 'just to look' has its place, but sight is most useful and works best in the context of actually doing something. The more precision demanded by the activity, the greater the benefit to the sight – always provided there is no strain.

Painting, drawing or model-making are all valuable, provided that concern for a finished result doesn't get in the way of a relaxed and enjoyable process. Colouring is a very relaxing pastime, a childish pleasure that gives crea-tive satisfaction even to those who would underrate their ability to paint or draw. It is an ideal activity in visual development; one is aware of the outlines, attentive to the scribbling motion of the pencil point and accepting of the result. The childishness of the task makes it easy for many adults to recapture a child-like spirit in their approach – exactly what's wanted.

In contrast, walking may not seem like a particularly 'visual' activity, until you try it with eyes closed. Hill-walking and climbing make constant demands on judg-ment through the vision, and give few opportunities for the staring daydream. Sailing and cycling, among other activi-ties, fall in the same category.

Ball games of all kinds have the same advantage; one is concerned primarily with hitting the ball, and clarity of vision does rather well from its secondary position. In a 'live ball' game such as tennis, the 'map' of the court in memory is the constant background to every decision and reflex action; the timing of every stroke requires perfectly relaxed concentration. The only pitfall is to be over-preoccupied with winning, as opposed to making the best of each shot. It is possible to play a surprisingly good game of tennis with relatively poor vision, provided it is approached in the right spirit. My game definitely improved when I first took off my glasses, which surprised me a little since I could barely see my opponent at the far end of the court.

In the teaching studio I constantly use games of catch, and juggling, to develop the focus of attention through an activity rather than on an object.

INTEGRATION AND BALANCE

Total or partial suppression of one or other eye, or big differences in acuity (anisometropia), suggest that, while the eyes may be individually fine, there is some misunderstanding between them and the brain. How is this to be overcome?

Working with separate eyes is helpful in any condition, provided relaxation is maintained. Here relaxation is vital. The basic strategy is to use the hands in a simple coordinated task, e.g. colouring, catching a ball, as a way of 'accessing' the two hemispheres of the brain, singly, in

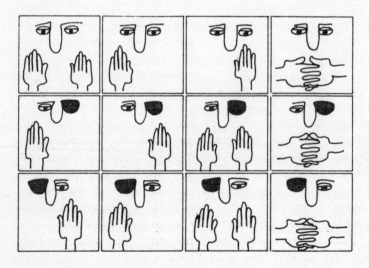

PERMUTATIONS OF HANDS AND EYES

rapid alternation, or together. If the eyes are also used separately and together this gives 12 modes (rapid alternation of the eyes is hardly feasible, and is not necessary). I must emphasise that both eyes are used equally and the total amount of time spent on one-eye work is quite small. This is much more helpful than the common practice of constantly covering the 'good' eye.

Working through the task in these permutations will show up any 'challenges', as inability, mental or physical discomfort, or excessive effort. The aim is to encourage free flow of energy so that the activity can be equally easy and relaxed in any mode. When this is the case it can be assumed that the relationship between each of the eyes and both of the brain hemispheres (and, accordingly, each other) is improved.

Muscle-testing techniques can accurately pinpoint and clear stresses, and may be the only way in some cases. For the most part, however, I prefer to work through the pupil's own experience, using flower remedies in the occasional sharp emotional reaction, but otherwise relying on conscious relaxation to allow the integration to take place.

In order to work with the eyes separately some means must be used to patch or occlude. Rather than cover the eye completely with a 'pirate patch', I prefer an open-sided shade that obstructs forward vision but maintains the peripheral vision. This can be done either with sunglasses which have had one lens removed and the other blacked out, or with the back of the hand (not the palm). The glasses are useful when the hands are required, as in ball games, but the back of the hand is favoured when swinging, or perhaps in drawing and colouring. The reason for using an open shade is that it encourages the peripheral vision of the obscured eye to integrate with the central vision of the unobscured one. This in turn enhances the central/peripheral integration of the open eye itself.

A final step to encourage integration is to split the field with a nose-card (or the hand – see opposite), creating the illusion indirectly of seeing two images. Integration and binocularity are only two sides of a coin, after all.

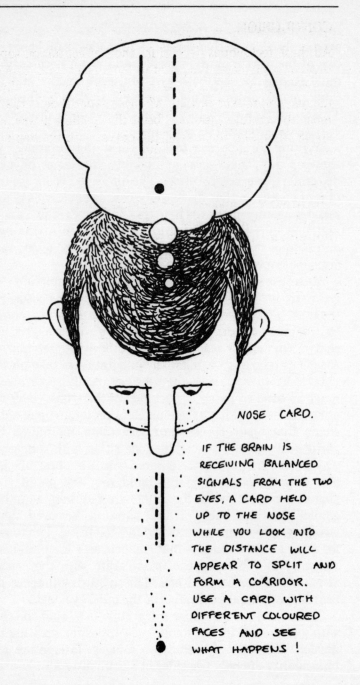

NOSE CARD.

IF THE BRAIN IS
RECEIVING BALANCED
SIGNALS FROM THE TWO
EYES, A CARD HELD
UP TO THE NOSE
WHILE YOU LOOK INTO
THE DISTANCE WILL
APPEAR TO SPLIT AND
FORM A CORRIDOR.
USE A CARD WITH
DIFFERENT COLOURED
FACES AND SEE
WHAT HAPPENS !

CONCLUSION

All these techniques depend for their effect not on sophisticated technology but on the intelligent and sensitive application of very simple principles. They are by no means foolproof or certain. My own experience is that the most successful cases have been those where I was, so to speak, flying by the seat of the pants, with no idea about what might happen and certainly no preconceptions as to what should happen. Conversely, cases approached with brimming confidence in my knowledge of 'what to do' have taught me valuable lessons. It all becomes less mysterious, but the fact remains that we are dealing not with a science but with an art.

9
STRANGE, RARE AND PECULIAR – A SELECTION OF CASES

Human beings are individual and so are their peculiarities of eyesight. Helmholtz's concept of bringing 'law and order to a mass of contradictions' has come close to creating an optical police state in which anomaly is criminalised. Some theory, some method, is needed in order to make sense of information and to investigate a situation but the investigation has to be done with an open mind and with respect for the individual's uniqueness.

Rather than rushing in to try and fix things, or even assuming that an aberration of sight necessarily needs fixing, our concern must be to find out what is going on. In the cases that follow, to the extent that the pupil and I have been able to find that out, we have succeeded and the improvement of sight has been a formality.

These are real cases, described from notes and recollection, fictionalised as much as necessary to ensure anonymity for these very special individuals who have taught me so much.

JOHN

John was a 15-year-old boy brought to me with a massive divergent squint, dating from his fourth year or so, which had resisted all attempts at treatment. I had never seen anything like it, but put on a brave face and set to work to teach the elementary procedures and see what came up. He learned to relax, he learned to see movement, he learned to appreciate colours, etc. But as we worked I realised that the biggest problem was the strategy that he had carefully developed over many years as a way of coping with the situation. I was fascinated to notice that this ran through into his use of language, which reflected a way of thinking that exactly paralleled the behaviour of his eyes. It was clear that whatever we might do, his way of thinking had to be fundamentally altered if we were to get anywhere.

He would talk about 'focusing'. It took a little while to establish that what he meant by this was making a massive effort to force his 'questionable eye' round the corner, so that he could ignore its image, temporarily 'curing' his double vision. 'Relaxing' was used to mean letting everything blur, with no direction of attention. His logic was bizarre – entirely consistent up to a point (he was highly intelligent as well as extremely likeable), but without warning would switch to a completely different point of view, remaining completely unaware of the discrepancy.

The lessons took on the character of seminars in semantics, and we went merrily round in circles while I abandoned any thought of getting the eyes to behave differently, instead concentrating on getting him to understand what I was talking about. One day he suddenly said 'Oh wait a minute, I get it', and as he spoke the eyes came together; possibly for the first time in his life he was seeing in a normal relaxed way through both eyes at once.

JANE

Jane was another high-spirited and highly intelligent teenager. For as long as anyone knew one eye had been so long-sighted as to be useless. She had none the less enjoyed normal vision, courtesy of her good eye, but this was now showing signs of developing myopia. Mother's first remark was 'We know you won't be able to do anything for the "lazy" eye, but we do hope you can do something with the good one.'

On investigation it turned out that the 'lazy' eye was totally suppressed, had distant vision of about 13/200 and could not see the reading type. The 'good' eye's vision was fluctuating between 20/15 and 20/20 – a little.'off', but no real problem. The strain of the unbalanced situation, together with increasing academic pressure, was obviously telling. Significantly, she liked drawing, but only from life – could not draw at all from memory. She liked music, could play the cello well, but had failed totally at the piano and hated it. It struck me that these were exactly the activities one would expect to be affected by poor brain integration. Her considerable intelligence also struck me as very left-brained, and rather brittle in the sense one associates with long sight. This was confirmed as we went to work.

'Now, if you look down the string, do you see one, or two?'

'One of course – why should there by two?'

'Because you have two eyes in different places.'

'Yes, but there's still only one, so why should I see two? That's STUPID.'

Good fun!

We debated the point at length over several weeks, and at a volume that quite alarmed neighbouring practitioners. One day, after a bout of metaphysical arm wrestling, she said slowly 'OK, I can see there should be two. So why can't I see them?'

The next week she caught a glimpse of two strings, and I sent her home to think about it. The next week we had done the impossible and obtained fully binocular vision, which she has retained since.

It was the same story with the swings. At first:

'I know they're still so why should they look as though they're still moving.'

But a month later:

'Of course it's moving. ANYONE can see that.'

'Some people don't.'

'Well they must be pretty stupid then!'

One day we were sitting in front of the test card discussing how the letters might move all by themselves. This idea was a bit much, and the debating society was in full swing.

'Yes but they can't move by themselves – I mean you've got to do something.'

'True. But the eyes will make little movements unconsciously if you let them.'

'But I still don't – UGH!'

'What's the matter?'

'They're moving. They're COMING OUT!'

Once over the surprise we shared a lot of fun watching the letters move. Working with this experience enabled the lazy eye to improve to about 20/30 for distance and to be able to read satisfactorily. The better eye was perfectly all right, and headaches were a thing of the past.

As each stage unfolded there seemed to me to be a corresponding change in personality. As the eyes began to work together and the strain was removed from the 'lazy' side, her intelligence, losing nothing of its edge, seemed to gain flexibility, to see more readily different sides to a question.

Her vision still has ups and downs; it is a vulnerable area, and in an intellectually and emotionally active teenager that is to be expected. The point is that she now works with her sight and not against it.

SONIA

The sight always reflects something of the general health, and conditions not thought of as visual at all can produce very powerful eye symptoms.

Sonia came to me on the off chance that I might be able to shed some light on an unusual problem. She had suffered for some time from ME – myalgic encephalitis, a loosely defined complaint involving fatigue and inflammation. Although it is a recognised syndrome, it is widely acknowledged that no two cases are alike. In this case the eyes seemed to be unusually involved. Sonia had been short-sighted for a long time, with no especial difficulties, but since the ME she found herself in a dilemma. She could not see without her glasses, but putting them on invariably caused an enormous aggravation of the ME symptoms, apparently inflaming every nerve in her body. She had tested this out quite carefully and was quite certain it was so.

This seemed to me to confirm very dramatically Dr Bates' point that poor sight involves nervous strain and that glasses add to it. In her weakened state, the added strain of the glasses was obviously being transmitted through her entire nervous system. We then found that bright light had the same effect, but that by gradually increasing exposure this reaction became more normal. Other work on the method produced improvement, both in her vision and her general symptoms.

To dismiss such a case as an anomaly, a freak, is to miss the point. The rare and extraordinary cases are different from the run of the mill not in kind but only in degree. By their intensity they highlight the features that are always present but easily overlooked in the less dramatic instances.

GEORGE

In the case of George, a newspaperman, physical discomfort was the only problem. At the age when one might expect presbyopia, failing sight, he retained perfect vision for all distances; however, the act of reading the printed word made him feel sick.

Learning to look in a relaxed way and sorting out a minor convergence problem largely relieved the symptoms, although not entirely. There were good grounds for suggesting a complete change of occupation, but this was not really on his agenda. Re-education, like politics, is the art of the possible.

MICHAEL

Presbyopia is a common complaint, but some people acquire it in uncommon ways.

Michael was a surgeon of late middle age, hoist with his own petard. Recovering from an anesthetic after a minor operation, he experienced a period of unpleasantly blurred vision and dissociation of the eyes. This is common enough, but usually clears very quickly. In his case, though, it persisted for a while, then cleared slowly, leaving him presbyopic and extremely put out since, before entering hospital, his perfect vision had given him great pride and satisfaction. And professionally he was faced with a dilemma; he could not work as a surgeon with blurred vision, but was conscious of the disturbance to his hand-eye coordination caused by glasses. He had the habit of working with his head close to the operation and, although he could see better from further away, it felt unsafe working like that.

He had no problems learning the work I set him, found it all fascinating, but began to get very despondent when he found the excellent results of the first few lessons hard to reproduce. He was obviously anxious to improve quickly and was prone to trying much too hard; the whole problem had obviously been triggered by straining to overcome his blur after the anesthetic. I pointed out that any improvement at all was better than 'inevitable' deterioration; that I was sure he would do better still, but that attitude was all important.

Like most presbyopes, he had problems with convergence as well as with accommodation, so, because of his anxiety to 'see' his progress, I took to measuring, on the string, his nearpoints in both aspects. His inclination was to push on through strain and discomfort to improve his score. However, gradually, I was able to persuade him to approach the exercise more passively, observing in a rather detached way the results of the process and making no effort at all. This would mean at times allowing the vision to blur or double and simply taking note of what he saw, all the while inhibiting his instinctive urge, which was to try and put it right. This seemed very strange to him, but when it became clear that his improvement depended entirely on the degree to which he put this peculiar philosophy into practice, he saw the point. Within a few weeks he was able to converge and accommodate accurately to about 6 inches with no strain at all.

He then began to comment that his vision was now excellent for reading material, but that he could not focus so well on other things, especially his work. I suggested that this would be because the print gave feedback that was less ambiguous than parts of people, but that he should practise looking at ordinary objects and working out how to make the same kind of mental connection. At work his possible nervousness about his responsibility and his need to see clearly would be a potential source of strain, so I suggested that he could practise on anatomical models to get the feel of the situation and gain confidence in his ability to see well in that position. He shortly afterwards reported that he was having no further difficulty.

The actual visual problem had been entirely routine and this very intelligent and open-minded man had been, if anything, more easily successful than most in using the techniques of vision improvement. However, the demands of his occupation had added to other factors and had created anxiety and impatience which could have undermined the entire process. His eventual success had required not only proper instruction in what to do, but considerable reassurance, encouragement and clear explanation, together with quantities of carefully chosen flower remedies – a time-consuming and arduous procedure for which both of us were richly rewarded.

JILL

The 'normal' refractive problems have the character of excessive stability. I have termed as 'chaotic' the conditions that arise from lack of stability, and which give rise to vision that changes too much and too often to be reliably corrected by lenses.

When Jill came to me she was more concerned about her sanity than her eyes. She had been severely short-sighted since her schooldays and she had, by herself, made the connection between her sight and a great deal of unhappiness that she had suffered at that time. Over the previous year or two her vision had become unstable, to the extent that if she had a pair of contact lenses prescribed, within a week they would be useless. An intrigued and extremely patient practitioner had given her 20 different sets of lenses in about as many weeks, then admitted defeat and referred her to a specialist who could tell her nothing about her condition but who had insinuated that she was neurotic. She needed to talk to someone who could at least help her make sense of what was happening.

The story sounded reasonable enough to me. I told her I had not seen a case like it before, but that it seemed perfectly intelligible that her sight was on the move, and even trying to correct itself, after years of restriction. It was the first time in the whole saga that anyone had attempted to give her an explanation, and there was immediate progress – after the first lesson the vision stabilised considerably, and in a short while the immediate problem was solved, basically by means of learning to relax and accept instead of fighting. A rather busy individual, Jill was not able to commit the time and energy I would have liked and, although working together threw up all kinds of fascinating insights, she was not really motivated towards abolishing her lenses altogether. A partial success then, but significant and worthwhile for all that.

MOLLY

The difficulty with near work associated with presbyopia has more to do with strain than with aging. When the vision is fixed in the mould of a particular habit, it will not respond freely to the current situation. As things 'free up', the vision may not necessarily improve but it will relate more appropriately to whatever is going on. This provides information that must be used to secure long-term improvement.

Molly was a charming and energetic lady of 30-something, deeply interested in languages and in fact studying Chinese in preparation for a working trip to the East. We were working successfully on her short sight when she suddenly brought in a new problem – she couldn't read. She wondered if stopping her being short-sighted had made her long-sighted instead? This of course is out of the question since the Bates work can only increase flexibility. On enquiring, it turned out that her exams had been brought forward by a whole month, and for the previous fortnight she had been studying every night to 3 am. I pointed out that this was a good way to create problems. She said she had often worked in a similar way before without any problems. I explained that previously her eyes would have been fixed by her lenses and not very responsive; now they were free to choose, they could more easily protest against their mistreatment. The relative unfamiliarity of the Chinese characters would be an additional source of strain. As it happened I could also recall an identical experience of my own in similar circumstances. We then practised some relaxed reading, first on English material, then on Chinese, identifying the additional strain and teaching her how to avoid it. That problem did not recur.

SUSAN

It is not necessary to *believe* in the method, just to be open-minded and do what is necessary. Totally negative attitudes obviously hinder progress. But, oddly enough, some people with such attitudes do take up the Bates method, apparently out of perverse desire to prove to themselves that nothing can be done. Even more strangely, some individuals experience considerable improvement without noticing or believing that is has happened. This seems to stem from the belief that nothing can be achieved without hard work; something as easy as the Bates method is therefore too good to be true, and therefore must be a catch.

Susan, an accountant, took a few lessons over a period

of months but was extremely concerned that she didn't have enough time to practise the exercises. In vain I protested that I wasn't giving her 'exercises' and I didn't care whether she practised or not, but that I did want her to listen to, and think about, what I had to say. She was adamant that she could not improve unless she practised exercises regularly and that there could not be any benefit from coming to lessons unless she did so. It was clearly a question of value for money.

The last time I saw her she had decided not to come again 'until she could find time to take it seriously.' Rather than debate the point, I agreed and then used the time to review the various things she had learned. I then took a quick test for reference and to my astonishment she tested 20/20 (her previous best had been 20/40). Although she agreed that she could see the letters quite clearly and read them several times, she was quite certain that her vision could not have improved because she had not been 'practising the exercises'. On the way out I established her legal fitness to drive with a selection of number plates at well beyond the required distance. She seemed puzzled, even put out, rather than pleased as we said goodbye.

JAMES

The belief in the need to do 'exercises' can be even more damaging when one *does* do them.

James called me one day with a real tale of woe. He had been told about the method by a friend who had lent him a book (I never did find out which book) that instructed him to do certain exercises and to leave his glasses off at all times. He left his glasses off and did the exercises (as he understood them), and here he was telling me that his vision was worse than before and that he now suffered from constant eyestrain and headaches. He could not even go back to glasses because they made matters even worse. What was he to do?

I told him to wear his glasses whenever he needed them, palm as much as possible and come and see me. It became obvious that he was constantly straining, even while palming, and it took a few months of regular visits to get to a 'normal' starting point for serious work. After that we progressed well, but his habit of introducing strain into even the simplest activity had to be watched every moment.

CHLOE

The degree to which emotional trauma is a factor in poor sight varies a great deal. While it is by no means always a main cause, in the cases where it does emerge it must always be faced, whether it is obvious at the outset or emerges indirectly through a more functional approach.

Chloe was a severely myopic 20-something, totally dependent on her contact lenses. She came for lessons infrequently but stuck to the method with astonishing fidelity, although with no more than glimmers of improvement in her vision. I have rarely been so close to saying 'Look, I don't think we're achieving very much here', but she was pleasant and cooperative, seemed to enjoy the lessons and was pleased at the thought of at least stopping her sight's rapid deterioration.

So I waited. Sometimes, out of the blue, an exercise would prompt her into telling me the most extraordinary things about her thoughts and feelings, and on these very clear indications I began to use the flower remedies. Then one day she came and told me that, while relaxing at home, she had experienced a completely clear 'flash', but that as it happened 'something inside me shouted NO!' I asked her what she thought this meant, and it triggered a stream of associations from her childhood, of repressed memories of things she was not allowed to see physically and metaphorically. In the remainder of that lesson we made as much progress with her vision as during the previous six months.

IAN

Sometimes the changes can be physical as well. Ian found that studying the method not only triggered a mental and emotional transformation: it actually re-arranged his face. As the tensions were shed from the eye muscles, the associated patterns in the facial muscles gave way too, leading to deep changes extending into the jaws, neck and shoulders, and all around the cranium.

His case was very extreme, but subtler forms of that kind of reaction are fairly common, pointing to the essential correctness of Dr Bates' hypothesis of the role of muscular strain, and the usefulness of associated work such as Alexander Technique and cranial osteopathy to increase the receptiveness of the entire physical structure.

JESSIE AND ALICE

The relationship between vision and general mental conditions becomes very clear when working with children, where one generally finds more direct response. Sometimes we deal with deep emotion, at other times just with bad habits. Exploring the visual facts of life is a productive starting point that will take us as far as we need to go, while avoiding over-involvement. The contrasted experiences of two nine-year-old girls show this well.

Jessie experienced a catastrophic lapse into myopia, so sudden and severe that it was obvious even to the doctors that glasses could not be the answer. It came out later that her family history had involved a succession of fairly serious upheavals, most of which she had withstood with extraordinary resilience until the death of a much-loved grandparent had proved the last straw. It seems likely now that her problem with her sight was reflecting her distress and symbolising a withdrawal into herself to sort things out, but at the time I was only able to guess at an unnamed distress. Rather than trying to normalise the sight I thought it best to prevent her developing unhelpful habits, as far as possible, so as to maintain the responsiveness of her sight and otherwise to wait on developments.

She became very interested in playing with strings and charts, but became really intrigued when I offered to teach her to juggle. Lessons fell into a pattern of 10 minutes' 'work', 40 minutes' juggling practice and 10 minutes' showing off to mum. At every visit her vision was noticeably better, and I began to wonder whether she could see perfectly well and was just coming for the juggling lesson – she even began to bring her friends.

At last there was no escaping it. She was seeing faultlessly, so I told her where to find a (cheap) juggling class. I was told later that just before her sight had returned to normal, she had experienced a remarkable series of dreams, which seemed to mark the resolution of her emotional problems. In this case the method played a supporting rather than a leading role, keeping the mechanism of sight, ready and prepared until she was able to use it. I consider it a great success.

Alice on the other hand, seemed to have nothing wrong with her except bad habits – slightly short-sighted (with a bias to one side) and steadily deteriorating. A common enough picture. The problem seemed to have started, as so often, in school, and her way of staring intently at anything she was unsure about made quite a picture.

It was interesting to see how quickly she responded. The problem had not been with her very long, and fortunately her mother had come to me instead of going for glasses. Everything we tried worked almost instantly. As soon as I explained the difference between straining to look and relaxing, she said 'Oh yes, I can see it all now', and promptly read the 20-foot line from that distance.

When it still seemed a little fuzzy we looked at the astigmatism, using a clock card. She said some of the lines looked a little blurred, and I suggested she use a knitting needle as a 'pencil with a rubber'. She promptly 'rubbed out the blurs and pencilled in the lines' until all the lines of the clock were equally clear, then treated the test card letters in the same way, whereupon her vision improved to 20/10. She was very taken with this new game and quickly worked out how to make her sight better or worse to order.

The Bates method can, of course, be learned at any age, but children around the ages of 7–12 perhaps have a special advantage in that they seem to be able to use a great deal of intelligence without allowing intellectual preconceptions to limit their trusting spontaneous nature. Adults have to learn, some more easily than others, how to recapture that spirit and use it to undo years of habit. Children are by nature truthful, and a child's sight always has important truths to tell.

CONCLUSION

Human beings are a diverse breed, and vision is a complex process. This book has described in outline an approach to visual problems based on the acceptance of that complexity and diversity.

The relationship between teacher and pupil requires balance, if not equality. The Bates teacher is not an expert handing down definitive wisdom, but merely has experience in the techniques and insight into the philosophy. The pupil however is always best placed to understand her own situation, and only from the growth of that understanding can come change. The teacher is a guide; one who knows the territory well enough to take charge of visiting explorers, to lead them to features of interest and to point out pitfalls until, finally, the explorers find their feet and begin to make their own discoveries.

But there can never be any guarantee. The saddest people in the world are those who refuse to attempt anything unless certain of success; who wish their teacher to be a packhorse, carrying them and their baggage all the way.

The happiest, and those who experience the greatest success, are those who are willing to take a chance and to allow 'getting results' to take second place to the interest and fun of experiencing the process. For those – and I have had the privilege of meeting many – anything is possible.

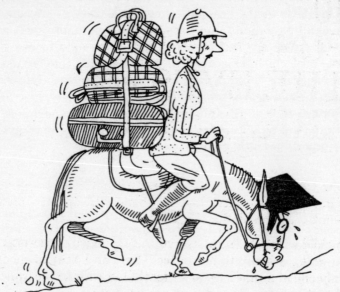

The saddest people ... are those who refuse to attempt anything unless certain of success; who wish their teacher to be a packhorse, carrying them and their baggage all the way.

10
POSTSCRIPT – THE EYES AS CHILDREN

Our eyes are children; they love us and wish to please. Kind words and attention fill them with joy; too many rebukes will break their heart.

A child wishes to learn, if anything, too much. The world is so wide, so many things to see. How can I bear to choose only one at a time? We must teach, but with forebearance, that the rule is one at a time – or none at all.

Call a child stupid, name it lazy. It will become so. Play is a child's work, the work of the eyes is the play of light – delight – a state of illuminated grace.

A child must be bold, go out and discover. We must encourage; teach wisdom, but not fear. Afraid to go, to touch, to look, afraid to see? Love conquers fear.

In all things important, all start equal. Those where we are unequal are unimportant. Don't ask 'Do my eyes serve me well?' but 'How can I ever repay what they have already done?'

If I am sad, my child will weep. Should I beat him for his sympathy, or should we console each other and find joy again together?

Children do not go wrong; what goes wrong is their relationship with the world. A word, a touch can put right so much.

When did you last hug your eyes?

TWO EXTRACTS

Since 1920 Dr Bates' book *Perfect Eyesight Without Glasses* has been available only in abridged form. The excised passages contain not only the details of his experimental work, which justify what might otherwise be taken as whimsical assertion, but also much of his most characteristic writing. These extracts are reproduced as giving a good indication of the character of the man and of his method.

PREFACE

This book aims to be a collection of facts and not of theories and insofar as it is, I do not fear successful contradiction. When explanations have been offered it has been done with considerable trepidation, because I have never been able to formulate a theory that would withstand the test of the facts either in my possession at the time, or accumulated later. The same is true of the theories of every other man, for a theory is only a guess, and you cannot guess or imagine the truth. No one has ever satisfactorily answered the question, 'Why?' as most scientific men are well aware, and I did not feel that I could do better than others who had tried and failed. One cannot even draw conclusions safely from facts, because a conclusion is very much like a theory, and may be disproved or modified by facts accumulated later. In the science of ophthalmology, theories, often stated as facts, have served to obscure the truth and throttle investigation for more than a hundred years. The explanations of the phenomena of sight put forward by Young, von Graefe, Helmholtz and Donders have caused us to ignore or explain away a multitude of facts which otherwise would have led to the discovery of the truth about errors of refraction and the consequent prevention of an incalculable amount of human misery.

REASON AND AUTHORITY

Some one – perhaps it was Bacon – has said: 'You cannot by reasoning correct a man of ill opinion which by reasoning he never acquired.' He might have gone a step further and stated that neither by reasoning, nor by actual demonstration of the facts, can you convince some people that an opinion which they have accepted on authority is wrong.

A man whose name I do not care to mention, a professor of ophthalmology, and a writer of books well known in this country and in Europe, saw me perform ... an experiment which, according to others who witnessed it, demonstrates beyond any possibility of error that the lens is not a factor in accommodation. At each step of the operation he testified to the facts; yet at the conclusion he preferred to discredit the evidence of his senses rather than accept the only conclusion that these facts admitted.

First he examined the eye of the animal to be experimented upon, with the retinoscope, and found it normal, and the fact was written down. Then the eye was stimulated with electricity, and he testified that it accommodated. This was also written down. I now divided the superior oblique muscle, and the eye was again stimulated with electricity. The doctor observed the eye with the retinoscope when this was being done and said: 'You failed to produce accommodation.' This fact, too, was written down. The doctor now used the electrode himself, but again failed to observe accommodation, and these facts were written down. I now sewed the cut ends of the muscle together, and once more stimulated the eye with electricity. The doctor said, 'Now you have succeeded in producing accommodation,' and this was written down. I now asked:

'Do you think that superior oblique had anything to do with producing accommodation?'

'Certainly not,' he replied.

'Why?' I asked.

'Well,' he said, 'I have only the testimony of the retinoscope; I am getting on in years, and I don't feel that confidence in my ability to use the retinoscope that I once had. I would rather you wouldn't quote me on this.'

While the operation was in progress, however, he gave no indication whatever of doubting his ability to use the retinoscope. He was very positive, in fact, that I had failed to produce accommodation after the cutting of the oblique muscle, and his tone suggested that he considered the failure ignominious. It was only after he found himself in a logical trap, with no way out except by discrediting his own observations, that he appeared to have any doubts as to their value.

Patients whom I have cured of various errors of refraction have frequently returned to specialists who had prescribed glasses for them, and, by reading fine print and the Snellen test card with normal vision, have demonstrated the fact that they were cured, without in any way shaking the faith of these practitioners in the doctrine that such cures are impossible.

[A] patient with progressive myopia ... returned after her cure to the specialist who had prescribed her glasses, and who had said not only that there was no hope of improvement, but that the condition would probably progress until it ended in blindness, to tell him the good news which, as an old friend of her family, she felt he had a right to hear. But while he was unable to deny that her vision was, in fact, normal without glasses, he said it was impossible that she should have been cured of myopia, because myopia was incurable. How he reconciled this statement with his former patient's condition he was unable to make clear to her.

A woman with compound myopic astigmatism suffered from almost constant headaches which were very much worse when she took her glasses off. The theatre and the movies caused her so much discomfort that she feared to indulge in these recreations. She was told to take off her glasses and advised, among other things, to go to the movies; to look first at the corner of the screen, then off to the dark, then back to the screen a little nearer to the center, and so forth. She did so, and soon became able to look directly at the pictures without discomfort. After that nothing troubled her. One day she called on her former ophthalmological adviser, in the company of a friend who wanted to have her glasses changed, and told him of her cure. The facts seemed to make no impression on him whatever. He only laughed and said, 'I guess Dr Bates is more popular with you than I am.'

Sometimes patients themselves, after they are cured, allow themselves to be convinced that it was impossible that such a thing could have happened, and go back to their glasses. This happened in the case of a patient ... who was cured in fifteen minutes by the aid of his imagination. He was very grateful for a time, and then he began to talk to eye specialists whom he knew and straightway grew skeptical as to the value of what I had done for him. One day I met him at the home of a mutual friend, and in the presence of a number of other people he accused me of having hypnotized him, adding that to hypnotize a patient without his knowledge or consent was to do him a grievous wrong. Some of the listeners protested that whether I had hynotized him or not, I had not only done him no harm but had greatly benefited him, and he ought to forgive me. He was unable, however, to take this view of the matter. Later he called on a prominent eye specialist who told him that the presbyopia and astigmatism from which he had suffered were incurable, and that if he persisted in going without his glasses he might do himself great harm. The fact that his sight was perfect for the distance and the near-point without glasses had no effect upon the specialist, and the patient allowed himself to be frightened into disregarding it also. He went back to his glasses, and so far as I know has been wearing them ever since. The story obtained wide publicity, for the man had a large circle of friends and acquaintances; and if I had destroyed his sight I could scarcely have suffered more than I did for curing him.

Fifteen or twenty years ago the specialist mentioned in the foregoing story read a paper on cataract at a meeting of the ophthalmological section of the American Medical

Association in Atlantic City, and asserted that anyone who said that cataract could be cured without the knife was a quack. At that time I was assistant surgeon at the New York Eye and Ear Infirmary, and it happened that I had been collecting statistics of the spontaneous cure of cataract at the request of the executive surgeon of this institution, Dr. Henry G. Noyes, Professor of Ophthalmology at the Bellevue Hospital Medical School. As a result of my inquiry, I had secured records of a large number of cases which had recovered, not only without the knife, but without any treatment at all. I also had records of cases which I had sent to Dr. James E. Kelly of New York and which he had cured, largely by hygienic methods. Dr. Kelly is not a quack, and at that time was Professor of Anatomy in the New York Post Graduate Medical School and Hospital and attending surgeon to a large city hospital. In the five minutes allotted to those who wished to discuss the paper, I was able to tell the audience enough about these cases to make them want to hear more. My time was, therefore, extended, first to half an hour and then to an hour. Later both Dr. Kelly and myself received many letters from men in different parts of the country who had tried his treatment with success. The man who wrote the paper had blundered, but he did not lose any prestige because of my attack, with facts upon his theories. He is still a prominent and honoured ophthalmologist, and in his latest book he gives no hint of having ever heard of any successful method of treating cataract other than by operation. He was not convinced by my record of spontaneous cures, nor by Dr. Kelly's record of cures by treatment; and while a few men were sufficiently impressed to try the treatment recommended, and while they obtained satisfactory results, the facts made no impression upon the profession as a whole, and did not modify the teaching of the schools. That spontaneous cures of cataract do sometimes occur cannot be denied; but they are supposed to be very rare, and any one who suggests that the condition can be cured by treatment still exposes himself to the suspicion of being a quack.

Between 1886 and 1891 I was a lecturer at the Post-Graduate Hospital and Medical School. The head of the institution was Dr. D.B. St. John Roosa. He was the author of many books, and was honoured and respected by the whole medical profession. At the school they had got the habit of putting glasses on the nearsighted doctors, and I had got the habit of curing them without glasses. It was naturally annoying to a man who had put glasses on a student to have him appear at a lecture without them and say that Dr. Bates had cured him. Dr. Roosa found it particularly annoying, and the trouble reached a climax one evening at the annual banquet of the faculty when, in the presence of one hundred and fifty doctors, he suddenly poured out the vials of his wrath upon my head. He said that I was injuring the reputation of the Post Graduate by claiming to cure myopia. Every one knew that Donders said it was incurable, and I had no right to claim that I knew more than Donders. I reminded him that some of the men I had cured had been fitted with glasses by himself. He replied that if he had said they had myopia he had made a mistake. I suggested further investigation. 'Fit some more doctors with glasses for myopia,' I said, 'and I will cure them. It is easy for you to examine them afterwards and see if the cure is genuine.' This method did not appeal to him, however. He repeated that it was impossible to cure myopia, and to prove that it was impossible he expelled me from the Post Graduate, even the privilege of resignation being denied to me.

The fact is that, except in rare cases, man is not a reasoning being. He is dominated by authority, and when the facts are not in accord with the view imposed by authority, so much the worse for the facts. They may, and indeed must, win in the long run; but in the meantime the world gropes needlessly in darkness and endures much suffering that might have been avoided.

THE SNELLEN TEST CARD

For more than 100 years the test card, an array of different-sized letters, has been the standard by which visual acuity is judged. Although it is used thousands of times daily in optical practice, very few patients, and by no means all practitioners, are really clear about its purpose.

The bottom line in measuring acuity is the ability to observe the presence of an object; another useful measure is the ability to distinguish similar objects. The limits of acuity in fact relate to the apparent size of an object, or, in more technical terms, the visual angle subtended by the object at a point on the retina. This angle is a function both of the object's actual size and its distance from the eye, and can be expressed in degrees and minutes of arc.

Hermann Snellen made his experiments to determine the limits of vision in people whose eyesight was generally acknowledged to be excellent – marksmen and so forth. He concluded that the limit of resolution for any individual feature would be a visual angle of 1 minute of arc (1'), and that distinguishing an object such as a letter required an overall 'size' of 5', with individual elements of at least 1'.

He therefore constructed a typeface on a square grid,

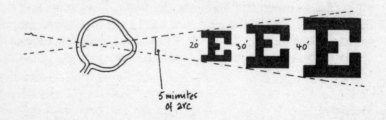

5 minutes of arc

arranging the shapes of the letters to fill the square as uniformly as possible. He eliminated letters that would not fit the scheme – W, for example, is never used in any test type – and decorated the letters with stylised serifs (cross-lines finishing off the strokes of the letters), which fill more of the square and aid discrimination between similar letters. All elements are kept to a uniform thickness both of line and, as far as possible, openings. Similarly, the spaces between letters are the same size as the letters themselves.

The prescribed distance for each line is that at which the optical angles correspond to 5' for the whole figure and 1' for the individual lines. Although Snellen calculated the limits of resolution from empirical data, recent research has shown that in fact 1' does represent the physiological limit for individual retinal cells. In practice it is possible to see more, and some people demonstrate fairly reliable vision at twice the normal limit, probably by a combination of mental image enhancement and the relaxed guesswork that is a part of all good seeing.

The normal test distance is 6 metres/20 feet. Cards are always calibrated beyond this point, old imperial cards have lines down to 10 feet while metric cards go to 3 or 4 metres.

When the card is used for testing vision it is important to be aware that it is not necessary, and may not even be physically possible, to read the bottom line. Most people assume that they are supposed to do so, and immediately begin to strain, making their vision much worse. Similarly, when the testcard is used for prescribing glasses, the commonly assumed aim is to try to achieve perfect vision for the bottom line. This is definitely wrong – by any standard all that can be required is adequate vision for the correct test line.

The combination of these two factors – worsening of the vision through strain and then over-prescribing through setting an artificially high target – is to make sure that glasses are prescribed to many people who have no visual difficulty and that, if there is a problem, the prescription is often twice as strong as necessary, leading to increased strain and accelerated deterioration.

It was a particular stroke of genius on the part of Dr Bates to realise that the instrument responsible for putting so many people into glasses could also be used to get them out. The essential purpose of the card is to give feedback; the clarity of the perception obviously corresponds to the performance of the eye in some way. If the information fed back is that the eye is not doing well, then this is likely to trigger the responses of anxious strain, resigned apathy, or an alternation of the two. This is what happens in most sight tests, allowing the vision to be fixed and measured in a defective state. If, instead, these responses are recognised, inhibited and replaced with a state of relaxed attentiveness it becomes possible to *use* the information to realise that the sight is variable, recognise the patterns of variation, and learn to steer them in the right direction.

It is relatively rare nowadays to find a Snellen-designed type in use by an optician, as the test cards have generally been superseded by 'modern' versions, the design principle of which is less clear. The British Standard types, for example, use a conventional typeface that has the advantage of familiarity, but which sacrifices the carefully built in 'identity tags' of Snellen's letters, and is less precise in the relation of line to space, while the letters are more closely spaced, as in a word. The overall effect of these differences is to make the type less legible. While this may make no difference – or even be an advantage – in refraction work, it reduces the reliability for acuity testing and the usefulness for improvement.

The Snellen-designed card adopted by Dr Bates includes numerals and geometrical shapes, both of which increase its sensitivity in testing and its usefulness for practice. In its 'negative' form – white letters on black – it becomes more useful still, since white letters remain visible (although distorted) at a distance, where black characters would blur into a haze. Reduced-size versions of the card are also very valuable for use at shorter distances – say 2–6 feet.

Transforming one's experience of seeing obviously involves a lot more than doing exercises with a test card, but as long as one's social usefulness is determined, as at present, by the ability not just to see, but to decipher signs and symbols, the test card, correctly used, will play a valuable part.

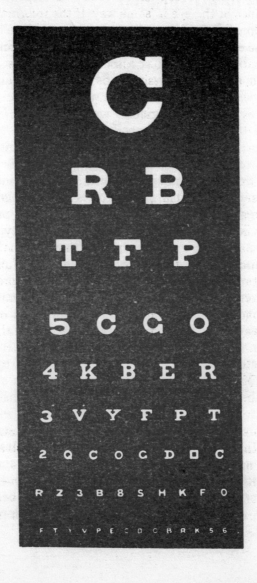

APPENDIX 1

CELLULAR LEARNING: A NEW LOOK AT THE THEORY OF EMMETROPIA

As stated in C 2, it is not necessary to assume that an eyeball needs to be strictly emmetropic in order for normal vision to be possible. It is a fact, however, that statistically, more eyes do grow towards the shape required for perfect vision (emmetropia) than would be expected if the process were entirely random, and it has therefore been assumed that there is a specific way in which the body regulates the growth of the eyes towards an emmetropic shape. From recent physiological research into the process of *emmetropisation* and its response to various influences in a number of animal species, it is becoming apparent that the growth of the eye is controlled by a physiological feedback loop (just as its behaviour, as we have seen, is controlled by a neuro-muscular feedback loop). In other words, learning takes place at the cellular level, in much the same way that we have described it taking place at the gross functional level. The mechanism seems to be that the clarity or otherwise of the image on the retina stimulates hormone secretions which accelerate or slow down the rate of growth of the eyeball, so controlling its axial length and hence focus. If weak (4d or less) spectacle lenses are placed in front of the eyes at certain stages in growth, then the development of the eye will change course to adapt to the altered condition. If the vision is completely disrupted, e.g. by fogging, constant darkness, constant light or strong lenses, the growth pattern goes haywire and the refraction becomes highly abnormal. Control populations which were not interfered with nearly all developed normal sight. This process has been convincingly demonstrated in chickens, tree shrews, and monkeys.

If this information is extrapolated to humans (which is presumably the ultimate point of such research), the consequence is obviously that Dr Bates was far more right than he ever knew: wearing glasses to 'correct defects' not only disrupts the functional development of vision, it actually perverts the development and growth of the eye away from normal. In principle, therefore, on the basis of this finding alone, no child should ever be given glasses as, left alone, the vision should normalise through the process of growth. In practice it will not be quite that simple: children are not chickens and, in particular, are more subject to the emotional disruption of vision so that the various benign interventions discussed throughout this book may be necessary to allow the process to normalise fully.

At the same time, this information suggests room for some revision to Dr Bates' theories and the practice of the method. For instance, the possibility of non-optical disruption of the hormone control mechanisms does make it more likely that the ordinary refractive errors, and such conditions as progressive myopia, *could* appear congenitally. Equally, however, it could be argued that the hormonal systems would in turn, in humans, be just as likely as muscular functions to be influenced by emotional states, so that in terms of prevention, and early diagnosis/ remediation the Bates approach would still be entirely viable.

In the case of remedial work with long term sufferers it might appear that a structural basis for the problem could limit the possibilities of improvement, or, at least, suggest that it could only take place over a long period, related to the cell replacement cycle, perhaps. That *may* be so, but it does not alter the fact that substantial improvements do take place, over a relatively short time span, so that this cannot be the whole story. The finding that small 'corrections' influence the growth of the eye can be used positively, as in the practice of using 'transitional' glasses, and progressively weakening the lenses in small steps so that the eyes gradually adapt. At the moment this process is used empirically by a few optometrists and others but it may be that the continuation of this kind of research, and its extension to human subjects, will suggest a rational and consistently useful way of planning such treatment.

A slightly more teasing question is, whether working at vision improvement on the functional level (if this involved improving clarity by refocusing congenitally ametropic eyes) might work against the process of emmetropisation (which depends on the blur in its natural state, so to speak, as its stimulus). Since, in practice, the improvements gained through vision education seem to become more rather than less stable over the longer term, for the moment, and until the position becomes much clearer, that is a risk I am willing to take.

Sources: research articles in *Vision Research* and in *Visual NeuroScience* 1994

MULTIPLE PINHOLE GLASSES

These notes have been compiled, and are now included here in response to many requests for information on this subject.

Background
Multiple pinhole 'glasses' have been in use for about thirty-five years. Slightly different versions have appeared on the market at various times and sometimes at excessive prices. The more expensive ones are generally better made and finished but there is no clear evidence as to whether the optical qualities are any different. Various claims have been made for their efficiency both as a visual aid, and as a means of improving unaided eyesight. Manufacturers often refer to the Bates Method in their promotional material and some have taken to supplying Dr Bates' book together with their product.

The general consensus among Bates teachers is that these devices are useful but that the claims sometimes made for them as a complete solution to visual problems, or as a replacement for, or improvement on, the **Bates Method** are exaggerated and misguided. The remainder of this chapter describes how they work and makes some suggestions for their use.

Optical principle

When an object is viewed through a very small aperture (*a pinhole*) a clear image will always be formed because only *coherent rays of light* are able to pass through, so that the 'blur circle' normally formed by an out of focus eye is reduced almost to the clear point that would be seen if it were in focus. This means that, provided there is no opacity of the eye or impairment of the retina, the object will appear clear regardless of any refractive error. The image through a single pinhole is very small and dim, but by using a regular array of similar sized holes it is possible to enlarge the field of vision and improve the overall brightness of the image while still retaining most of the clarity of at least the central area.

In practice, the holes are of course rather larger than an ideal pinhole (which would be infinitesimally small!) and the size of hole is a compromise between clarity of resolution and brightness of illumination. Similarly, in theory the lens material should be infinitesimally thin (and at the same time perfectly opaque); in practice most versions are rather thick so that the light travels through a 'tunnel' with rather unpredictable optical results.

Visual Effect

The initial experience for most people is of a form of 'insect vision', with distinct but multiple images overlapping in rather a confusing way. Every movement gives rise to a pronounced flicker which many people find quite disturbing at first. Some complain of increased strain and headaches at first use. This indicates that some manufacturers' claims that the eyes 'automatically' relax when using these things are a touch over-enthusiastic. Rather, as with so many other beneficial things, *you have to find out how to relax in order to be able to use them*, which some find easier than others. The flicker of movement must be just accepted – the Bates Method has a lot to say about the experience of visual movement – and after a while it becomes possible to find a way of centralising a particular object so as to eliminate the multiple images, at least from the central area. When this can be done the central object becomes noticeably clearer than its surroundings which is a useful demonstration of Dr Bates' principle of *central fixation.*

Advantages for Vision

According to Dr Bates, wearing glasses adds to the strain which underlies poor vision: however, until one learns more relaxed ways of using the eyes, simply taking glasses off can also make matters worse. Since when wearing pinhole specs the dioptrics of the eye are irrelevant, it follows that at the very least one can be freed from the need to conform to the pattern of strain for which the glasses were fitted, while enjoying vision sufficiently clear to largely eliminate the urge to strain to see better. This does not in itself promote improvement, but reducing the 'need' to strain and the time spent wearing glasses, increases the chances of success by other means.

It is fundamental to the Bates approach that vision is a constant learning process based on the *feedback of information* between eyes and brain. The traditional Bates practices are designed both to increase the sense of contact with what is seen and the awareness of variations in vision. This line of thought is developed further by at least one manufacturing company who design their holes to *limit* rather than *eliminate* the 'blur circle'. The idea is that at the worst the vision is good enough to make it easy to maintain *relaxed interest* and to improve the basic flow of information, but that it is possible for improved function to bring about noticeable improvement so that there is also a flow of feedback about the behaviour of the eye (which would not be so with true pinholes): in this way the eyes are constantly encouraged and good behaviour is rewarded. This idea is certainly plausible and broadly in agreement with Dr Bates's principles.

The multiple array encourages two important aspects of normal visual behaviour, *shifting* and *centralisation*. In turn it is found that these can only be achieved if the use of the eyes is basically *relaxed*.

Various Uses

In general the use of pinhole glasses is two fold: as a developmental tool in vision improvement, and as a straightforward substitute for glasses in certain situations.

They can be freely used as a substitute for glasses in any situation where they are found to give adequate vision, although *not* for driving or any other potentially hazardous activity. Generally they will be easier to use in good light than poor. It is possible to use them for visually static tasks like TV and computer use as they are much preferable to glasses since they encourage more mobility in the eyes, but not everyone finds this feasible.

In Bates or other vision improvement work it may be very good to try various practices, such as swings and chart exercises, alternately using the pinholes and unaided, rather than using the pinholes exclusively.

One possible drawback of the multiple pinhole array is that it will often be impossible for the two central sight-lines of a person's eyes to be perfectly aligned on a single object through two corresponding holes. This makes it impossible to have normal binocular vision with normal convergence and probably accounts for many of the experiences of strain and headache reported by a few users. Many versions of the 'glasses' however come with removable lenses and this can be very helpful. If one of the lenses is removed, the relatively clear vision from the 'pinholed' eye can be integrated with the unobstructed field of the other, avoiding the convergence problem and giving rather good vision overall. If this is done for short periods alternating the eyes it may also encourage better vision in the unassisted one. Work with alternate single eyes is used a great deal in the Bates Method, commonly using 'patching glasses' with a blacked-out 'lens'. This can be enhanced by having one eye blacked out and the other 'pinholed'.

Suppliers: Trayner Pinhole Glasses make good quality 'glasses' £25–30.

Visual Arts are developing vision training kits which will include pinhole systems. Sae for details (address as Bates Association).

PRK (PHOTOREFRACTIVE KERATECTOMY)

One of the major developments in the medical treatment of poor sight over the last twenty years has been surgical modification of the cornea – radial keratectomy. Originally developed in the USSR, this had been hailed as a miracle operation, enabling the normalisation of sight in a few minutes of surgery. PRK adapts the basic technique to the use of computer guided surgical lasers which promise quicker and more accurate treatment (the advertisement claims normal sight in five seconds), and with fewer complications.

The reasons for mentioning it here are:

- It has been suggested that this is more satisfactory than the Bates Method with 'all those exercises': this is an idea I would like to discuss.
- Many people have written to ask for my views: here they are.

PRK seems to appeal to people who dislike wearing glasses but lack the motivation to do personal work on their vision. The reasons given for preferring PRK to, say a course of Bates lessons are generally:

- Bates lessons are expensive
- Bates teachers do not guarantee results
- Bates work demands a certain personal commitment, practice and so on.

on the other hand:

- PRK, although quite expensive, is a 'one off' investment with a reliable outcome
- PRK is 'done for you' and does not require the same personal effort.

Straight away, we can say that the cost of PRK for both eyes (currently £700–1000) would buy an awful lot of Bates lessons and a few good dinners, and if you have read this far you will, hopefully, have realised that the workload involved in the method is not necessarily all that great.

As for PRK, whether it is simple, reliable and undemanding depends on the point of view. Personally, I do not much like the idea of subjecting the most sensitive part of the body to a burning tool (a laser is, after all, only a high-tech blowlamp), and I find it odd that people who will express grave qualms about exposing the eyes to ordinary sunlight should think that this is OK.

For an unbiased view, however, let us look at what the people who practise it have to say. The college of ophthalmologists publishes a patient information document[1] which all intending patients are required to read, and on that basis, to sign a declaration that they have been fully informed of all risks and limitations of the procedure and freely consent to it, waiving many possible rights and claims.

According to this document:

- Treatment *to within one dioptre of expectation* may be achieved in eyes with a myopic refraction of 1–6 dioptres (i.e., most people who have the operation will still not have normal sight).
- The greater the degree of myopia the greater the penetration of the laser needed and the greater the chance of corneal scarring: intermediate myopia of 7–12 dioptres may be treated but with a greater chance of significant regression, and of increased corneal opacification and with a danger of lasting corneal scarring (i.e., the worse your vision is and the more you are likely to want the operation the less good an idea it is).

- Immediate post-operative pain may be severe but is moderated by ointment and pain relief tablets (i.e., it hurts).
- The healing process varies from patient to patient and may take many weeks or months before it is complete and the second eye can be treated (i.e., it may go on hurting for a long time).
- Vision may be blurred for 3–6 months (i.e., blurring which in some cases cannot be overcome even by spectacles).
- Treatment of the first eye will cause a difference of focus between the two eyes, necessitating contact lens wear in the unoperated eye.
- About 80% of eyes heal in a predictable fashion leaving 20% with a less certain outcome which may include overcorrection or regression (i.e., for one in five people it doesn't work at all).

In other words: the procedure, although quick in itself is likely to lead to a period of at least six months of disturbed vision and considerable discomfort, at the end of which one eye only may have 'normal sight', in which case the process can be repeated, or may not, in which case the patient will be left indefinitely with the eyes out of balance.

It is no wonder then that a long list of those unsuitable for treatment includes:

- Those who are inappropriately motivated or do not comprehend the rationale of treatment (i.e., anyone who will be dissatisfied if they do not, after all this, obtain normal vision).

The statement patients are required to sign includes the following:

- Surgical results ... cannot be guaranteed.
- Certain side effects are possible ... (including) cloudiness, irritation, subsequent long sight, persistent short sight.
- It is understood that the list of complications is not

complete (i.e., the practitioners bear no responsibility for *anything* that may happen as a consequence.

- I understand that ... it is essential that I attend all follow up visits and adhere to the taking of all recommended medications (these include antibiotics, steroid drops, painkillers).

The college also publishes practice guidelines for surgeons which take an even more cautious view.

One study quoted indicates that, of 38 eyes treated in the range −1.75/−5 D, 92 per cent achieved correction in the range +/−1 D.S. The highest proportion actually achieving normal sight (i.e., not needing glasses at all) was 50 per cent. A more detailed study shows that below −6 this was likely to worsen to 25 per cent.

Bear in mind that the reference is to eyes, rather than patients: if the chance of an eye being corrected to normal is only 50 per cent, the chance of one patient having both eyes corrected to normal must be rather smaller than that.

An interesting article in *Optometry Today*[2] discusses the question fully and concludes:

'Optometrists should not defend eyeglasses and contact lenses for their own sake. Patients don't come to OD's office for eyeglasses or contact lenses, but rather for good vision. If there's a way to safely provide that to some patients more conveniently ODs owe it to patients to deliver that to them.

'ODs also need to let go of the academic idea that anything less than 20/20 is unsuccessful correction. Many doctors sniff at the fact that excimers can only get within 1.00 D of emmetropia. Patients who are currently −7.00 D myopes would love to be able to see well enough to find their alarm clock, their glasses or contact lenses.'

... to all of which one can only say 'amen'. Whether that gives this risky, expensive, and not quite trouble-free procedure a real advantage over vision education is another matter which I lead the reader to judge.

On the other hand, the feasibility of this technique, with all its uncertainties, points to the equal feasibility of what Dr Bates proposes. It is obvious that the changes of axial length of the eye required to correct the vision are very small, since only tiny amounts of tissue are removed. (The text book illustrations of the elongated myopic eye are enormously exaggerated). That being so, only very small variations in the muscle balance will be needed to produce the same result, so why not do it that way and leave the eyes intact?

References

1   College of Ophthalmologists 1993
    Excimer Laser photorefractive keratectomy
    Patient information document
    Best clinical practice guidelines
2   *Optometry Today* – Insight: 'Will PRK with excimer lasers eliminate spectacles?'

USEFUL
ADDRESSES

THE BATES ASSOCIATION

The Bates Association of Great Britain exists 'to advance the knowledge and practice of the methods of visual re-education developed by and named after the late William H. Bates MD'. Its main functions are at present:

- To act as a professional regulatory body.
- To encourage and facilitate contact between teachers.
- To regulate the training of teachers.
- To act as a source of public information about the method.

There is no facility at the present time for non-teaching membership, but contact with those who are interested and would wish to support the work is always welcome.

A register of teachers is produced and regularly updated. All teachers work mainly in private practice, teaching through individual consultation; some additionally lecture, give group workshops, accept residential pupils for intensive tuition or train student teachers.

All enquiries should be accompanied by a stamped self-addressed envelope, and should be addressed to:

The Secretary
The Bates Association of Great Britain
PO Box 25
Shoreham by Sea BN43 6ZF
Sussex

RELATED DISCIPLINES

Alexander Technique
STAT
266 Fulham Road
London SW10 9EL
0171 351 0828

Bach Remedies
The DR Bach Centre
Mount Vernon
Sotwell Wallingford
Oxon OX10 OPZ
01491 839 489

Homeopathy
Society of Homeopaths
2 Artizan Road
Northampton NN1 4HU
01604 21400

Kinesiology
Kinesiology Federation
Box 7891
London SW19 1PA
0181 545 0255

Health Kinesiology
Jane Thurnell-Read
12 Castle Road
Penzance
Cornwall
TR18 2AX
01736 64800

Edu-K-creative vision
c/o Kay McCaroll
14 Golders Rise
London NW4 2HR
0181 202 9747

Bates Kinesiology
c/o Anthony Attenborough
128 Merton Road
London SW18
0181 874 7337

OVERSEAS

Bates Method and related vision improvement work
International contact is limited at present and the work
offered in different countries may differ substantially or in
detail from UK practice.

Australia
Janet Goodrich
Natural Vision Improvement
Cabooltre
PO Box QU 4510

Belgium
Mme Agliy Mathot
133 Rue Grosse Lenberg
BT7 1180 Brussels

Germany
Wolfgang Gillessen
Ettal Str 42a
8000 Munchen 70

Wolfgand Hätscher-Rosenbauer
Obergasse 16
D-6118 Bad Vilbel
Tel: 06101-6933

USA
There are currently estimated to be around 50 teachers of
the Bates work in the US.

The Bates Teachers' Association
c/o Jerri-Ann Taber
Vision Training Institute
11303 Meadow View Road
El Cajon
Cal 92020

The Bates Teachers' Association maintains a list of
teachers in all states and information on opportunities for
teacher training.
  The Vision Training Institute offers teacher training in
a number of modes including a three month intensive
programme and a correspondence/video course.

Rosemary Gaddum Gordon
Cambridge Health Associates
355 Broadway
Cambridge
Mass 02139

Dr Marilyn Rosanes-Berrett
510 E 89th Street
New York
NY 10028

Self-healing work incorporating vision improvement

Meir Schneider Centre for Self-healing
1718 Tarawal St
S Cal
CA 94116

Martin Brofmann
2067 Broadway Suite 27
New York
NY 10003

BIBLIOGRAPHY

BOOKS ON *THE BATES METHOD*

Generally available in UK
W.H. Bates, *Good Sight Without Glasses*, Faber, reprinted as *Better Sight Without Glasses*, Grafton Books.

Aldous Huxley, *The Art of Seeing*, Chatto & Windus, 1941, reprinted by Granada.

Jonathan Barnes, *Improve Your Eyesight*, Angus & Robertson 1988.

Robert-Michael Kaplan, *The Power Behind Your Eyes*, Inner
Traditions, 1995.

Robert-Michael Kaplan, *Seeing Without Glasses*, Beyond Words Publishing Inc. 1994.

Christopher Markert, *Seeing Well Again Without Your Glasses*, C.W. Daniel.

Dr Marilyn B. Rosanes-Berrett, *Do You Really Need Eyeglasses*, 1990, Pulse.

Out of print books (OP) – enquire at libraries
Foreign publications (Imp) available from
specialist booksellers
W.H. Bates, *Perfect Eyesight Without Glasses*, Central Fixation pub co., 1919. OP Reprinted 1991: Health Science Press, P.O. Box 70, 8349 Lafayette Street Mokelumne Hill Cal. 95245 Imp.

Emily Liermann: *Stories From the Clinic*, Central Fix. pub. co, 1926, OP.

Margaret Darst Corbett, *Help Yourself to Better Sight*, Prentice Hall, 1949 reprinted Melvin Powers Imp.
How to Improve Your Sight, Faber, OP.
Quick Guide to Better Vision, Prentice Hall OP.

Dr R.S. Agarwal, *Mind and Vision*, School for perfect eyesight, Pondicherry Imp.

Dr R.S. Agarwal, *Yoga of Perfect Sight*, School for perfect eyesight, Pondicherry Imp.

B. Gayelord Hauser, *Better Eyes Without Glasses*, Faber, OP.

C.S. Price: *The Improvement of Sight by Natural Methods*, Chapman & Hall, 1953, OP.

Books on the eye and vision
Helmholtz, *Treatise on Physiological Optics*, reprinted Dover Books.

May & Worth, *Diseases of the Eye*, Bailliere Tindall & Cox, 1906–1950, OP.

D.D. Michaels, *Visual Optics and Refraction*, University of California, 1985.

R. Brooks Simpkins, *The Basic Mechanics of Human Vision*, Chapman & Hall, 1939, OP.

R. Brooks Simpkins, *New Light on the Eyes*, Vincent Stuart, 1958, OP.

R. Brooks Simpkins, *Oculopathy*, Health Science Press, 1963, OP.

R. Brooks Simpkins, *Visible Ray Therapy*, Health Science Press, OP.

Books on the Alexander Technique
Chris Stevens, *Alexander Technique*, Vermilion.

Wilfred Barlow, *The Alexander Principle*, Gollancz.

F.M. Alexander, *Man's Supreme Inheritance*.

F.M. Alexander, *Constructive Conscious Control of the Individual.*

F.M. Alexander, *The Use of the Self.*

F.M. Alexander, *The University Constant in Living*, Gollancz.

Books on Homoeopathy
Dr Nelson Brunton, *Homoeopathy*, Vermilion.

Samuel Hahnemann, *Organon of Medicine*, UK edn Gollancz.

J. Compton Burnett, *Curability of Cataract*, Imp.

J. Compton Burnett, *Delicate, Backward, Puny and Stunted Children*, Imp World Homoeopathy Links, New Delhi.

Catherine Coulter, *Portraits of Homoeopathic Medicines*, North Atlantic Books, (2 vols) Imp.

The Bach Flower Remedies
Dr E. Bach, *The Twelve Healers*, C.W. Daniel.

Dr E. Bach, *Heal Thyself.*

Mechthild Scheffer, *Bach Flower Therapy*, Thorsons.

Peter Mansfield, *Flower Remedies*, Vermilion.

Books of General Relevance
Olive Brown, *Your Innate Power.*

Louise L. Hay, *You Can Heal Your Life.*

Jacques Lusseyran, *And There was Light*, Floris Books, Edinburgh.

Jacques Lusseyran, *The Blind in Society/Blindness: a new seeing of the world.* Proceedings no 27 Myrin Institute, 521 Park Ave. NY Imp.

John Cassidy and B.L. Rimbeaut, *Juggling for the Complete Klutz*, Fontana (The Waldorf School, Adelphi University, Garden City, NY).

Meir Schneider, *Self Healing: my Life and Vision*, Arkana.

Meir Schneider, *Manual of Self Healing*, Viking Penguin.

M. Scott Peck, *The Road Less Travelled*, Rider.

M. Scott Peck, *People of the Lie*, Simon and Schuster.

Many people also derive useful insights from the books, too numerous to mention, of Krishnamurti, Gurdjieff and Carlos Castaneda.

INDEX

Page numbers in *italic* refer to the illustrations

Other natural remedy titles available from

VERMILION

ALEXANDER TECHNIQUE

An introductory guide to
the technique and its benefits

Chris Stevens

This guide to the Alexander Technique concentrates on the method itself, seen from the student's viewpoint. In a straightforward way, it answers all your questions about the technique and provides background information on its development.

The author is an experienced teacher of the Alexander Technique and has written an informative and instructive guide for all those interested in learning the technique and how it works.

AROMATHERAPY

An introductory guide to
professional and home use

Gill Martin

This revised and updated guide to aromatherapy has been written to answer all the common questions that the consumer and practitioner of other related therapies often ask. Gill Martin, a practising aromatherapist, is well aware of the particular concerns of first time patients and defines who it can benefit and how to find the right practitioner.

She also provides illuminating background information on this increasingly popular treatment and discusses the experience from a patient's point of view.

REFLEXOLOGY
An introductory guide to
its uses and how to find a practitioner
Anya Gore

This consumer's guide to reflexology concentrates on the treatment itself, as seen from the patient's point of view. It answers in a clear and direct way the most common questions asked about this therapy, such as how to go about finding a practitioner and what kinds of problems it can treat.

Anya Gore, a practising reflexologist, also provides background information to this increasingly popular treatment.

IRIDOLOGY
A guide to iris analysis
and preventative health care
Adam J Jackson

Iridology is an ancient diagnostic technique which uses analysis of the iris of the eye. It is a painless, non-invasive and astonishingly accurate method of health analysis, which reveals the condition of every organ in the body.

Iridologist Adam J Jackson explains in a straightforward way how iridology works, and provides a guide to self analysis.

MASSAGE THERAPY
A complete introduction to the technique and benefits of massage
Adam J Jackson

A natural, safe and extremely effective therapy for everyone, massage can be used as an aid to training in sport, in promoting healing after an injury, or as a relaxation technique.

This comprehensive introductory guide to massage is ideal for all those considering treatment.

A-Z OF NATURAL HEALTHCARE
Belinda Grant

This informative and comprehensive guide to natural healthcare lists a range of therapies detailing a wide variety of approaches, methods and treatments.

All the therapies share a view of the individual as being more than simply a physical body, and that the integrity of all parts of a person is central to their health. This book is a complete and up-to-date compendium of natural medicine for everyone.

FLOWER REMEDIES

Peter Mansfield

Flower remedies are a wonderfully simple and totally safe way of helping the body to fulfill its natural tendency to be healthy. Working on an emotional level, these remedies have the effect of making you 'feel better'. They stimulate the body to overcome the causes of physical illnesses and recover its equilibrium. In this way the remedies also complement other traditional or alternative healing methods.

To order your copy direct from Vermilion (p+p free), use the form below or call our credit-card hotline on **01279 427203**.

Please send me

...... copies of **ALEXANDER TECHNIQUE** @ £6.99 each

...... copies of **AROMATHERAPY** @ £6.99 each

...... copies of **REFLEXOLOGY** @ £5.99 each

...... copies of **IRIDOLOGY** @ £8.99 each

...... copies of **MASSAGE THERAPY** @ £7.99 each

...... copies of **FLOWER REMEDIES** @ £7.99 each

...... copies of **A-Z OF NATURAL HEALTHCARE** @ £5.99

Mr/Ms/Mrs/Miss/Other (BlockLetters)

....

Address...

....

....

Postcode................................Signed................................

HOW TO PAY

☐ I enclose a cheque/postal order for £......................... made payable to 'Vermilion'

☐ I wish to pay by Access/Visa card (delete where appropriate)

Card Number ☐☐☐☐☐☐☐☐☐☐☐☐☐☐☐☐☐

Expiry Date ☐☐☐☐

Post order to **Murlyn Services Ltd, PO Box 50, Harlow, Essex CM17 ODZ.**

POSTAGE AND PACKING ARE FREE. Offer open in Great Britain including Northern Ireland. Books should arrive less than 28 days after we receive your order; they are subject to availability at time of ordering. If not entirely satisfied return in the same packaging and condition as received with a covering letter within 7 days. Vermilion books are available from all good booksellers.